What T
"Ve...

"Dr Lansing and Colonel Quist have performed a great public service by writing a book that not only speaks directly to our veterans affected by PTSD but also to others including family and loved ones involved with their recovery." Well done!

GENERAL JOSEPH RALSTON
USAF (Retired), Former Supreme Allied Commander, Europe, NATO.

"Powerful! Every page is shattering! Such a need for this to be public! Many thanks."

MAC GIMSE ("MAXIMUS"), PHD
Professor Emeritus, St. Olaf College, Northfield, MN.

"This book is a revelation of unknowable magnitude. This needs to be shoved in the face of every service member and spouse. But more importantly, it needs to be shown to the public and explained to the children that suffer unknowingly and unintentionally. This is written in a way that puts an upbeat, easy reading tone on a very serious and quite tragic subject. And as I lived through some of the things spoken about in the book, it's perspective of the follow on generations of service members is a dialogue that often does not happen. The value of this book for future generations is impossible to quantify ... this is fantastic, thank you for everything you're doing."

SERGEANT JASON SWOFFORD
US Marine Corps retired (2/5 F Company, Ramadi Iraq 2006-07; 1/5 B Company, Nawa District Helmond Province Afghanistan 2009-Purple Heart, WIA).

"An exhaustively researched and compiled tome on a most timely subject written by authors who truly know whereof they speak—highly recommended reading for all who are affected by this serious societal problem."

COLONEL DAVID J. MARTINSON ("DOGFACE")
USAF (RET); BA, MA, MBA, PHD
Retired Professor of Shakespeare.

"A comprehensive and much needed assessment of veterans in crisis, those who have returned from military combat to their hometowns in America but who have been unable to shake the devastating effects of war. Our family knows. Our grandson, a seriously wounded purple heart combat Marine who put his life on the line in Iraq and Afghanistan is one of so many vets whose civilian life has been throttled by PTSD."

PETER F. "GUS" CHARLSTON
BA, MA; Professor of Humanities and Ancient Greek Tragedy, Portland Community College; Steering Committee & Education Director, Classic Greek Theatre of Oregon.

Steve Lansing, PhD, LICSW and Colonel B. Wayne Quist, USAF Retired, both Vietnam veterans, set out to create a book to inform veterans of the nature of the disorder, illustrate its manifestations throughout recorded history, encourage them to seek professional treatment, and provide suggestions to keep from falling into an attitude of hopelessness and despair. The book is not intended as do-it-yourself therapy. It is, instead, an awareness and knowledge builder with the goal of getting the PTSD sufferer to seek professional help. The document is replete with references to resources in the community and national organizations for support in the veteran's journey to wholeness. Having myself treated veterans with PTSD for many years in the VA, I highly recommend this book.

GERALD D. OTIS, PHD
Las Cruces, NM

"Veterans In Crisis" will certainly give encouragement to PTSD victims in need of understanding. Understanding goes two ways: the ones who are afflicted and those who suffer for their dear ones. We can personally relate to that. Our son endured extended and intense medical horror as a teen, and even after three decades, time has not healed all wounds. Mental and emotional and physical scars do not heal. This book's comprehensive analyses will be a valuable resource for legions of PTSD sufferers and caregivers."

RHODA VAN TASSEL
BA CHAPMAN UNIV., MA UNIV. OF IOWA
Retired Art History and Humanities Instructor at Palomar College, CA. Active in community theater productions.

Well done! "Veterans in Crisis" narrates the impact that combat has in causing serious trauma and how it greatly affects our soldiers' emotional and physical health. Let's help them heal!

CHRIS JAMES HEISE, MSW, LICSW
Alliance for Healing, 4505 White Bear Pkwy #1500, White Bear Lake, MN 55110.
www.alliance4healing.com

"For thousands of years, mankind has evolved innumerable new ways to kill their fellow man, yet the one constant has been the human being. The impact of battle over time on the human condition has been constant, though not well discussed, until now. With this work, the effect on a soldier, being placed in the carnival of blood trying to kill and not be killed, is traced through history. Likewise, our understanding, or lack thereof of the impact this has on the person, is also shown. It is hoped that this study, Veterans in Crisis, will open up to those living with, or helping those who have, PTSD understand they are not unique nor somehow flawed but rather one of the human race who has seen the angry face of combat and rightly felt its impact upon their psyche and thus guide them on a path to an easier life."

MARC STORCH
Historian and researcher who proudly worked with those who served.
Madison, Wisconsin

Veterans in Crisis is a must read, mandatory issue, for all combat veterans and those who have been in a combat zone. Combat veterans know the people looking out for them are going to be fellow veterans who understand what it means to have been on the tip of the spear. Civilians cannot fathom what a combat veteran has experienced, and expressing it only makes things worse. This work can help civilians understand a little better. Written from the mindset of a military manual, it can be opened randomly to any page and read piecemeal when time or necessity requires it. This is the type of work any GI is familiar with.

SHANE CHRISTEN
Veteran author, lecturer, military museum curator, Red Wing, Minnesota.

VOLUME TWO

VETERANS IN CRISIS

JOE'S STORY
Untreated Trauma in a Decorated World War II Veteran

By Dr. Steve Lansing
& Colonel B. Wayne Quist

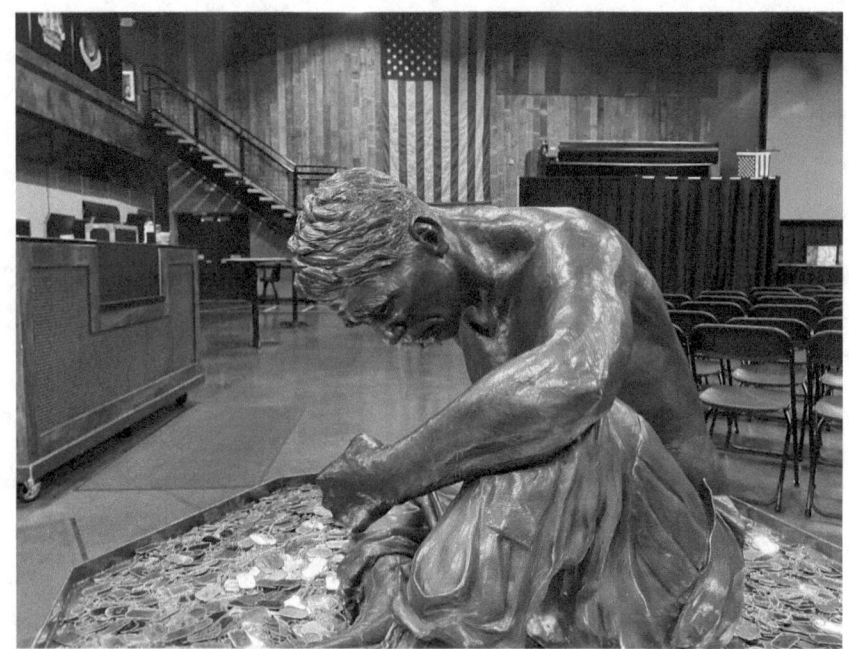

"Silent Battle" Bronze Warrior courtesy of Eyes of Freedom, Grove City, Ohio.

MISSION BIG WILLY-WON

POST-TRAUMATIC DEATH–GROWTH–REBIRTH–LIVING–DYING–GROWING AGAIN

"Traumatized people chronically feel unsafe inside their bodies: The past is alive in the form of gnawing interior discomfort. Their bodies are constantly bombarded by visceral warning signs, and, in an attempt to control these processes, they often become expert at ignoring their gut feelings and in numbing awareness of what is played out on the inside. They learn to hide from their selves."

– BESSEL A. VAN DER KOLK, M.D.
"The Body Keeps the Score."

VETERANS EMPOWERED INC
Treating the Unique Needs of Those Who Served

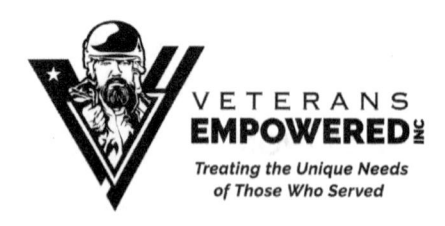

Copyright© 2024 by Veterans Empowered, Inc., a Minnesota 501©3 nonprofit corporation, established to educate and inform veterans, care providers, and the public about post-traumatic stress disorder (PTSD). No part of this book may be reproduced, stored in an electronic retrieval system, or transmitted electronically in any form or by any means without the prior written permission of Veterans Empowered, Inc., the authors, and publisher, except for reviewers who may quote brief passages to be published in a newspaper, magazine, journal, or electronic media.

The information and advice contained in this book are based upon the research and the personal and professional experiences of the authors. Neither the publisher nor the authors are engaged in rendering professional advice or services to readers or users of this book, in any of its paper or electronic issues or formats. The information, ideas and suggestions contained in this book are not intended as a substitute for consulting with your physician, trauma trained mental health professionals or any other related medical providers.

Neither the authors, Veterans Empowered Inc., nor the publisher of this book, in its various media formats and versions, shall be liable or responsible for any loss or damage allegedly arising from any information or suggestions contained in this book. This book is not intended as a substitute for professional trauma therapy. Instead, our intent is twofold: (1) Our goal with the general population is to inform and educate others about PTSD and how the impact of trauma can influence the lives of those individuals who have experienced such events. (2) For those suffering from PTSD, know that you are not alone in this battle and that countless others are there to support you; the stigma that may have been pointed toward you is something that warriors returning from combat have experienced since the beginning of history.

Volume Two of "Veterans in Crisis:"Joe's Story" highlights Joe's PTSD and was first published in 2010 by Brown Books Publishing Group, Dallas, TX under the title "God's Angry Man: The Incredible Journey of Private Joe Haan" by B. Wayne Quist.

First printing 2024

Volume Two Hard Cover ISBN: 979-8-218-49986-0
Volume Two Paperback ISBN: 979-8-218-48169-8

Cover Design by Aaron Ferguson and Kirsten Berg

Printed in the United States of America

CONTENTS

Suffering Makes Men Think 1

A Life of Hard-earned Wisdom 7

God's Angry Man 15

The Trauma of Private Joe Haan 23

The Orphanage 32

Indentured on a Farm 39

On the Road 46

CCC Camp 47

A World at War 61

After the War 104

High Steel 106

Evenings With Joe 129

A Symposium with Joe 141

Joe's Epilogue 153

Acknowledgements 163

Articles of Incorporation 166

Sources and References 171

The Authors 189

DEDICATED TO FELLOW VETERANS WHO SUFFER FROM PTSD

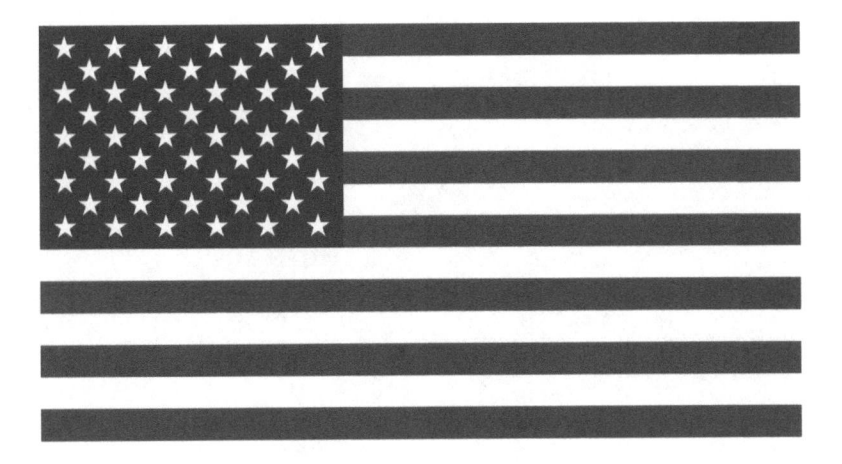

THE ESSENCE OF TRAUMA:

Overwhelming
Unbelievable
Unbearable

"There are only two ways to live your life. One is as though nothing is a miracle. The other is as though everything is a miracle."

-ALBERT EINSTEIN

Volume Two

JOE'S STORY

"Suffering makes men think.
Thinking makes men wise."

—JOE HAAN

IN MEMORY OF
JOE B HAAN
PFC US ARMY WORLD WAR II
FEB 26 1918   JAN 7 1992
SILVER STAR
BRONZE STAR MEDAL
PURPLE HEART

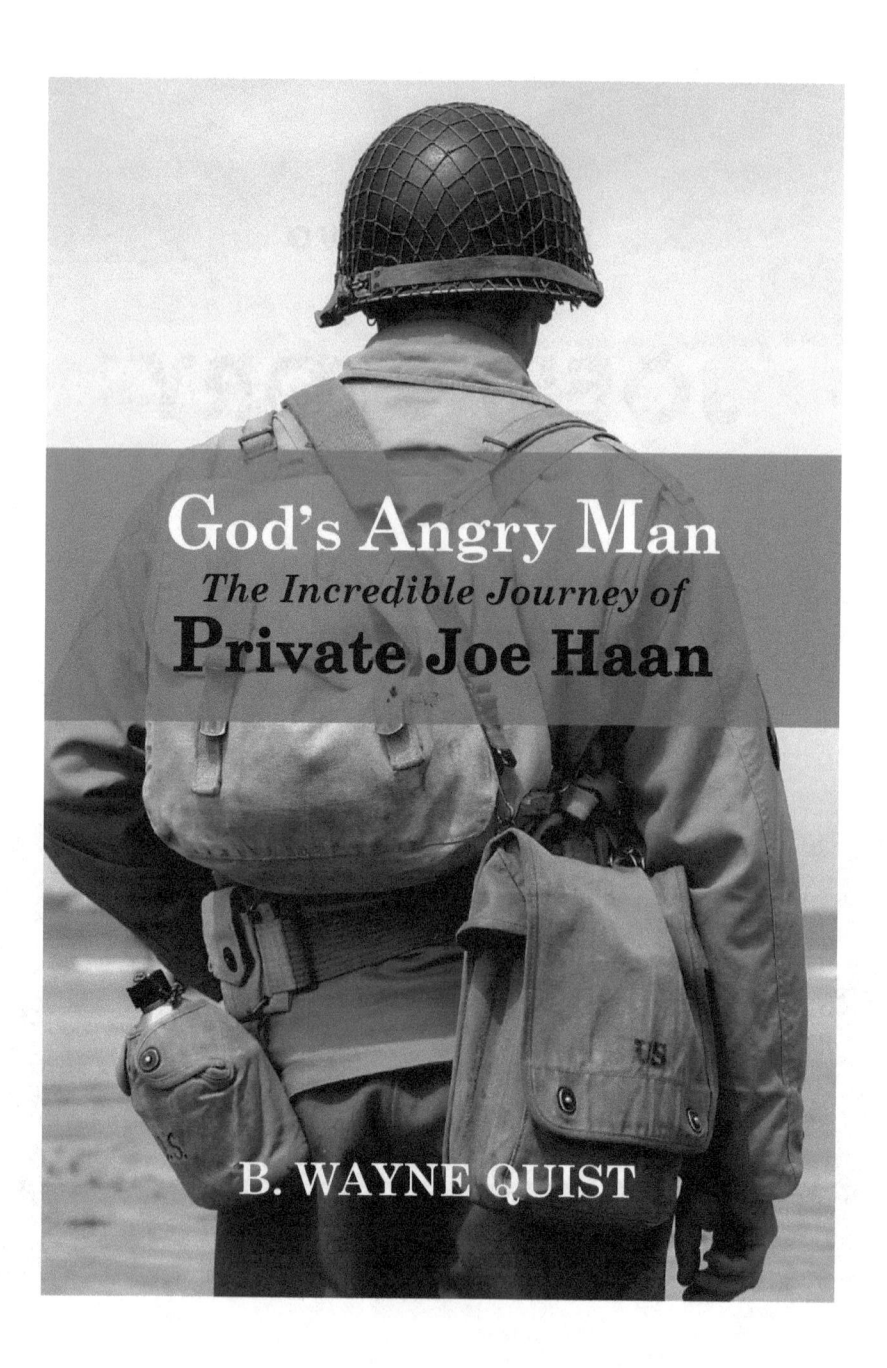

God's Angry Man
The Incredible Journey of
Private Joe Haan

B. WAYNE QUIST

God's Angry Man achieves exactly what we strive to do at The National World War II Museum: to tell the story of the war through the eyes of those citizen soldiers who were there. Through his Uncle Joe's eloquent letters, poems and other writings, B. Wayne Quist has given the reader a unique perspective on the war that changed the world.

—GORDON H. "NICK" MUELLER, PHD
President and CEO, The National World War II Museum
New Orleans, Louisiana

MINNESOTA POET & AUTHOR GARRISON KEILLOR:

Garrison Keillor Wrote:

"Private Joe Haan was a Minnesota boy who endured the unendurable and emerged a great man. A poet and musician, a Purple Heart hero of WW II, and a self-educated man who from rose the bleakness of the Great Depression. This is a book of hard-earned wisdom."

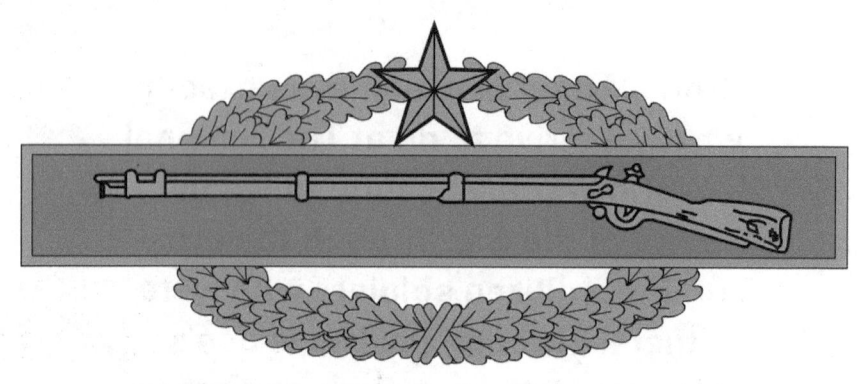

- Silver Star for gallantry in action.
- Silver Star and Bronze Star medals for valor behind German lines in Battle of the Bulge.
- Wounded in hand-to-hand combat 1945, decorated with Military Order of the Purple Heart.

Joe's Story

"THERE IS NO AVOIDING WAR.

IT CAN ONLY BE POSTPONED TO THE ADVANTAGE OF YOUR ENEMY."

NICCOLÒ DI BERNARDO DEI MACHIAVELLI

ITALIAN DIPLOMAT, AUTHOR, PHILOSOPHER AND HISTORIAN.

BEST KNOWN FOR HIS POLITICAL TREATISE *"THE PRINCE."*

WRITTEN ABOUT 1513, PUBLISHED 1532.

TO BE EMPOWERED, THE DOC SAYS...

Veterans in Crisis

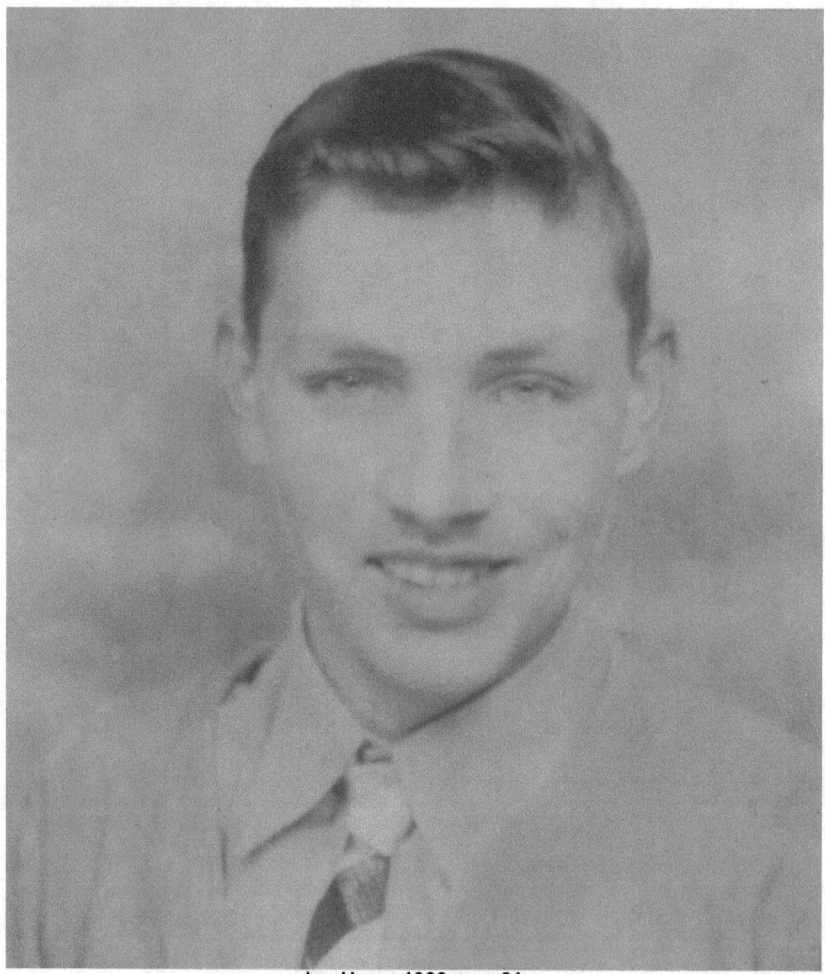

Joe Haan, 1939, age 21.

A LIFE OF HARD-EARNED WISDOM

"I have seen the pain in Joe's eyes when he talked about his father or mother, the Orphanage, the war." – Joe's friend Tim Carlson

- The story of a common man with uncommon vision and uncommon experience.
- Told thru 50 of Joe's surviving poems, essays & songs.
- Written from 1938-1990, autobiographical commentary.
- Stark, gut-wrenching, self-revealing.
- Joe told the truth as he saw it.
- Traumatic death of his mother at age 7.
- Trauma of the Owatonna Orphanage.
- Trauma on a farm, indentured to a cruel, sadistic farmer.
- Self-education during the Great Depression.
- Riding the rails around the country with bums and hoboes.
- CCC Camp, one long boot camp preparing for war.
- A Private soldier in Patton's Third Army in Europe, while facing some of the toughest fighting in World War II.

Joe wrote his classic poem, *"Memories of Death,"* as he waited to die, sharing a foxhole with a dead German soldier for three days in Alsace, France, November 1944, just before the Battle of the Bulge.

THE INCREDIBLE JOURNEY OF PRIVATE JOE HAAN

"Sometimes man is so completely confounded by the enigma of life that he attempts to escape into a cocoon of myth and falsity, never to emerge into the light of knowledge."

—Joe Haan, Notebook I – "The Last Iconoclast"

Nothing about Joe Haan's life was "easy." With little formal education, Joe taught himself everything he knew. Through his struggles, he was the ultimate survivor—growing up poor in St. Paul, forgotten in a lonely orphanage, living a slave's life indentured to a cruel southern Minnesota farmer, serving as a private soldier during some of the toughest fighting in World War II.

For nearly ten years after escaping from the hated German farm, Joe was on the move. He rode the rails in boxcars with hobos and bums during the Great Depression, slept under the stars in the great North Woods as part of the Civilian Conservation Corps, and crouched in muddy foxholes as a member of Patton's Third Army. Joe never slowed, and he never stopped fighting. Throughout it all, he coped with his trauma by becoming remarkably self-educated and expressing himself through his poetry, stories, and music.

Joe's life was an extended crucible—a constant fight for the survival of the fittest. He was the ultimate survivor, like a primeval animal in the wild, stalking his next meal. Few were better at it than he was, for out of necessity Joe developed keen insights, intuition, and instincts. He informed himself in many fields of knowledge—from astronomy, archeology, poetry, and philosophy to farming, fishing, trapping, steelwork, and taxidermy. Like Leonardo, Joe was a "disciple of experience," and he was a survivor.

Joe was a man who firmly believed that to live, to survive as a species, mankind must adapt and evolve in what he called the cosmic shooting "gallery of life." Joe was appalled at the persistent tyranny of human stupidity, the ignorance that plagued the world. To Joe, chief among these tyrannies was organized religion, and he railed against authority from his earliest days. He was quick to temper and sometimes solitary. But he was also artistic, poetic, and had a dry wit. In his final days, Joe proudly proclaimed to everyone why he was truly "god's angry man."

"Joe's Story" was composed and stitched together from Joe's old letters from the 1930s and 1940s, historical documents, war records, Joe's Army files, and recollections of Joe's friends and relatives. Together, these materials paint a portrait of *"god's angry man."* The language of the narrative captures Joe's spirit; the poetry and letters are pure, unadulterated *Joe Haan*, straight from his combat-damaged soul to his pencil and paper.

This is a true story of a Minnesota boy consigned at the age of seven to the infamous Owatonna Orphanage and indentured as a virtual slave to a cruel German immigrant farmer for eight long years during the Great Depression. Joe's PTSD and his writings, based on the latest research into post-traumatic stress disorder, demonstrate the therapeutic value of art and poetry.

When Joe finally escaped the brutality and trauma of the farm, he rode freight trains around the country from 1936 to 1939 and soon discovered free public libraries in every city across America. That's where he learned to read and write and keep a journal to express his inner feelings and to find release. Joe's story is a biography of trauma, told through Joe's gut-wrenching poems and essays.

Coming out of eighteen months in a CCC camp along the Canadian border in late 1941, Joe enlisted in the Army immediately after Pearl

Harbor and emerged from the war a decorated hero from Patton's Third Army in Europe. He was nominated for the Silver Star for Gallantry, awarded the Bronze Star Medal for Valor and the Purple Heart when wounded in hand-to-hand fighting with two fanatical young Nazi soldiers. At war's end, Joe helped liberate a Nazi concentration camp in Upper Austria near the German border with Czechoslovakia.

Joe's haunting poem "*Memories of Death*" echoes his trauma. It was written in the fall of 1944 just before the Battle of the Bulge and describes Joe's conflicting emotions about the German people, feelings of hatred first formed on the farm. But when he was trapped for three days in the same foxhole with a dead German soldier, expecting to die himself, Joe came to realize that both he and Corporal Friedrich Hofmann of the German Wehrmacht were common victims of tragic circumstance, that here was a young man like himself, trapped in war.

Joe wrote in his journal from France in 1944: "*I wondered if those at home whom we represented here in this mud would ever realize and appreciate what mental anguish and physical torture we, their infantry, were living through, with only one thought uppermost in our minds, to survive.*"

Later, while guarding German prisoners of war in 1945, Joe wrote of the trauma of war in his poems "*Guard Duty*" and "*Soldier's Lament:*"

> A violent thing I do today,
> In futile battle men I slay
> Who have been but a year and a day
> In time that here they had to stay.

After the war Joe became a fearless union ironworker in Houston, Texas walking and bending high steel for 33 years, erecting skyscrapers and reciting his poetry at noon lunch breaks. Joe hated violence and social injustice, and on his last day on the job before retiring, Joe wrote a classic poem, **"High Steel,"** in tribute to his fellow ironworkers.

> *In all the world of adventurous men,*
> *The high steel boy is one of them,*
> *On gird or truss or bridging high,*
> *Many a man has had to die.*

Throughout his life, Joe loved to recite his poetry, as well as other materials he had memorized over the years. His writings vibrate with the tell-tale signs of PSTD, and his poems are enhanced when read aloud. Everyone who knew Joe remembers his lively recitations and commentary, especially when he was motivated with a little beer or wine, which was always present in the evenings after work.

When we would visit Joe in Houston over the years, he would invariably start his evening discussions—they were really extended lectures or monologues—by talking about the *"big picture"* of life and the lessons of survival he learned along the road of hard knocks he had traveled from 1918 to 1945.

Joe's *"Survival Lesson"* is a good introduction to Joe for he firmly believed that to live—to survive as a species—mankind must adapt and evolve as new challenges are faced in the *"cosmic shooting gallery of life."*

We owe a special thanks to the trauma pioneers who have helped the world better understand and counter the destructive effects of PSTD. We owe James Haan, Joe's son, a special debt of gratitude for saving Joe's poems, art collections, notes, and war materials and for carrying on the spirit of Joe in his daily life.

Veterans in Crisis

TO BE EMPOWERED, THE DOC SAYS...

JOE LOVED MARK TWAIN

"I NEVER LET MY SCHOOLING INTERFERE WITH MY EDUCATION."

"MARK TWAIN" (SAMUEL LANGHORNE CLEMENS 1835–1910)

AMERICAN WRITER, HUMORIST, ENTREPRENEUR, PUBLISHER AND LECTURER, THE *"GREATEST HUMORIST THE UNITED STATES HAS PRODUCED."*

WILLIAM FAULKNER CALLED MARK TWAIN, *"THE FATHER OF AMERICAN LITERATURE."*

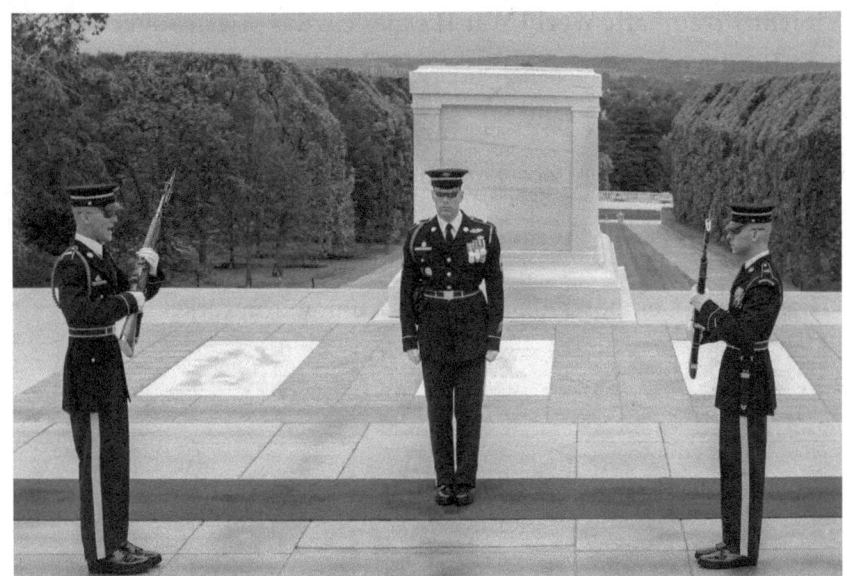

Tomb of the Unknown Soldier, Arlington Cemetery

A LIFE OF TRAUMA AND SURVIVAL

Alcoholic father, premature death of an angelic mother.

Institutionalized — drab and loveless orphanage; stern, bleak-eyed matron, Miss Morgan.

Daily trauma—indentured teenage farmhand; abused for eight long years.

"Slave to ignorance" on a small, remote Minnesota farm; lack of love, thirst for knowledge, little formal education.

Escape from brutality on farm, rode freight trains around the country with depression-era tramps and hobos, working odd jobs—one long boot camp.

Security in Roosevelt's Civilian Conservation Corps (CCC) camp in Minnesota North Woods.

Violently traumatic World War II experience as private soldier in Patton's Third Army.

Conflicting emotions while sharing a foxhole with a dead German soldier for three days in Alsace-Lorraine, France, October 1944.

"Memories of Death." Written in a foxhole in France.

"High Steel." Composed on last day as a union ironworker.

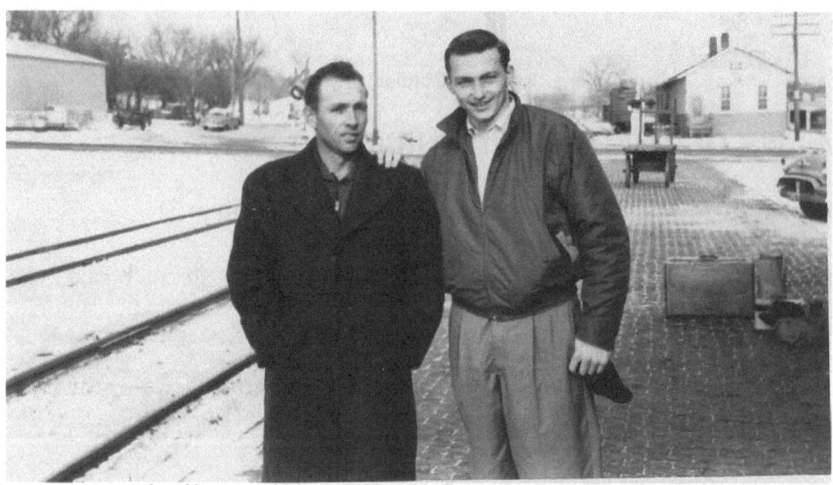

Joe Haan and his nephew, Air Force Lt. B. Wayne Quist, at Northfield, MN train depot, April 1959

"GOD'S ANGRY MAN"

- Orphaned, Indentured, Self-Educated
- Thinker & Teacher
- Workingman's Poet
- Paleontologist & Evolutionist
- Philosopher & Stargazer
- Geologist & Artist
- Professional Taxidermist
- Silver Star Combat Infantryman
- Career Union Ironworker

Joe had shown his inability to accept discipline at the orphanage, and it got worse on the German farm. But in CCC camp and the Army the rules and regulations were more strictly enforced. And there were plenty of dumb sergeants and brainwashed officers in the Army. This was especially true in Patton's Third Army under combat conditions. No one screwed up or mouthed off and got away with it under General Patton.

One of Joe's problems was when he took a drink of anything containing alcohol. After a few beers or a little French Sauterne wine, Joe was ready to take on the entire battalion or tear into his own sergeants for the slightest perceived offense. This is exactly what he did during his unit's much needed rest in Metz, France, shortly before the Battle of the Bulge. That's when Joe was demoted to Pfc for the last time and was reassigned from the artillery to the front lines of Patton's infantry.

Joe left the Army in November 1945 with the same rank he had following boot camp—Private First Class (Pfc), one stripe on his sleeves. During nearly four years in the Army, Joe was promoted to Corporal (two stripes) at least three times. Some of his Army records are missing, and he may have been promoted to Corporal four times and even Sergeant (three stripes) for a short while. Even so, he was always busted

Veterans in Crisis

back to his favorite rank of Pfc, mostly for fighting and insubordination. Joe left the Army at the end of the war with 16 months of combat service and nearly four years' active service as a highly decorated private soldier.

Joe remembered standing inspection in Germany toward the end of the war when the inspecting general saw the Purple Heart and Bronze Star Medal on Joe's chest, along with his other combat awards and medals for expert marksmanship. The general asked why Joe hadn't been promoted, and the captain said Joe was a better soldier as a private. The general looked at Joe and smiled. He understood.

Joe's buddies said he was a shining star that brightly illuminated their surroundings wherever he went with his songs and poetry. They also said Joe epitomized what was later called the *"Greatest Generation"*— World War II veterans steeled and molded by the hardships of the Great

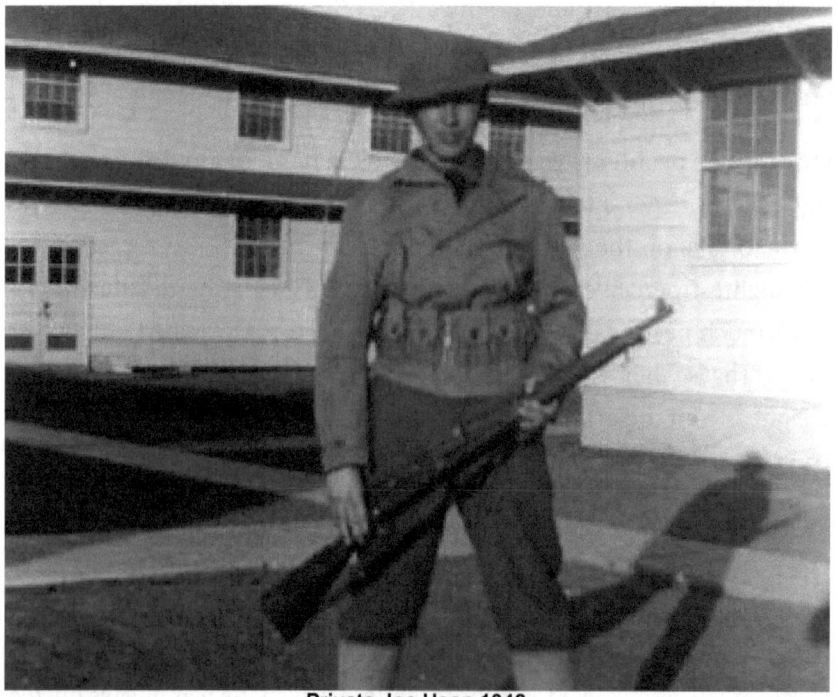

Private Joe Haan 1942

Depression. In Joe's case, he was also molded by the early death of his mother, the orphanage, his lonely existence on the hated German farm, riding the rails with hobos, and near death at the remote CCC camp.

Joe landed on Utah Beach and reached the front lines with Patton's Army in August 1944. Goaded on by anti-German Army propaganda, he was ready to kill *"Krauts"* to get even with the hated farmer and his German accent—until he spent three days in the same foxhole with the corpse of 18-year-old Corporal Friedrich Hoffman and recognized the common bonds of humanity and the futility of war. The experience triggered Joe's poem, *"Memories of Death."*

Joe's story is based on his journals and chronology of Army service from surviving military records, wartime letters, notes Joe kept while in the Army, and unit histories Joe received over the years from fellow veterans, compiled from war records for their reunions.

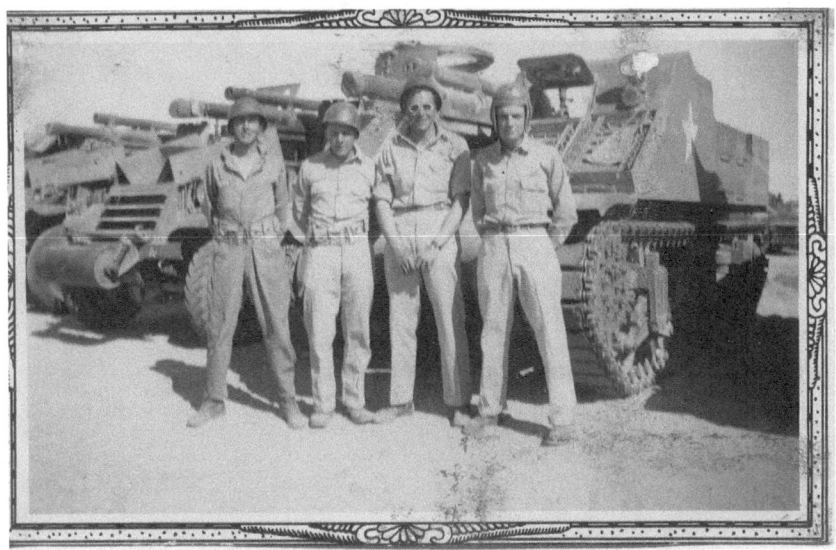

Private Joe Haan, 1942, training with tank destroyer company.

Veterans in Crisis

ERNIE PYLE 1943

"I Love the Infantry."

The troops loved Ernie Pyle, especially the dirty, grimy, cold, grunt riflemen in Patton's Third Army.

"There Are No Atheists in the Foxhole."

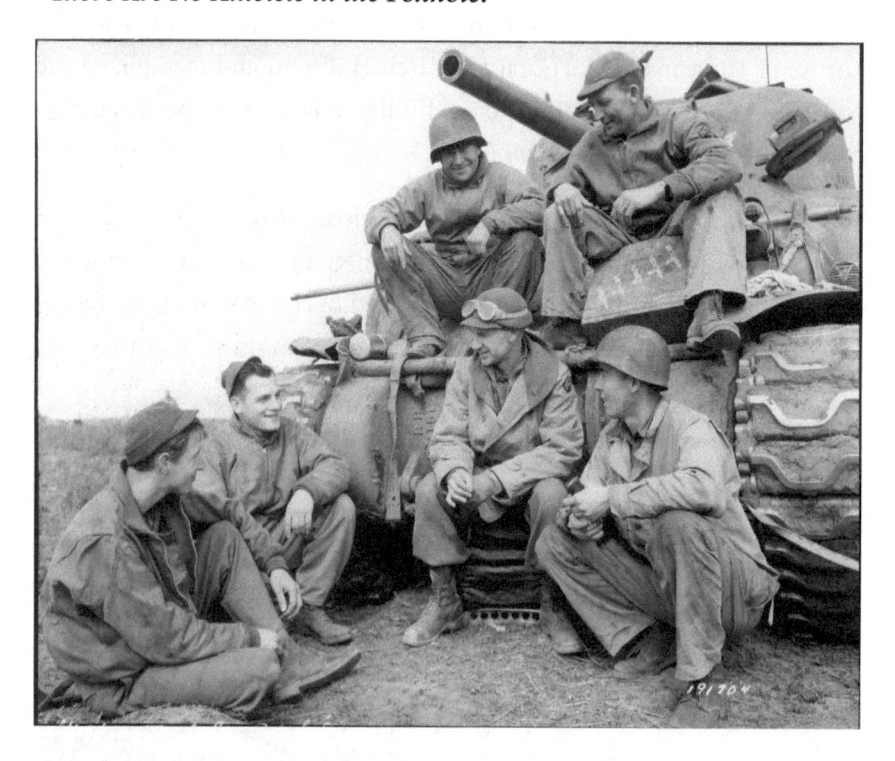

"No war is really over until the last veteran is gone."

Joe's Story

THE BEGINNING OF WISDOM IS WHEN WE START TO LEARN THE DIMENSIONS OF OUR IGNORANCE.

TO BE EMPOWERED, THE DOC SAYS…

Veterans in Crisis

*"It ain't what you don't know
that gets you into trouble.
It's what you know for sure
that just ain't so."*

MARK TWAIN

*"Knowing yourself
is the beginning of all wisdom."*

ARISTOTLE 384-322 BC

*"Knowing others is intelligence;
Knowing yourself is true wisdom."*

LAOZI
*ancient Chinese philosopher, author of The Tao Te Ching,
contemporary of Confucius 551 BC – 479 BC*

PARADISE DISORGANIZED

By Father Fa-nang-ler, Ex-Soul Trapper

I just returned from paradise,
What I observed shocked my eyes.
No method or manner have they there,
And no one really seems to care.
I asked the keeper of the gate,
"What's the population rate?"
"My good man, god only knows,
We have them stacked, unnumbered rows."
I then inquired whether a quota be,
He raised his staff for me to see,
"You see there, high up in the sky—
Room enough for all to die."
Sir, may I enter the glittering room,
And see the precious golden throne?"
"Oh, no! And never, earthly friend,
That's reserved for haloed men."
So, what fools we mortals be,
To be snared in a heavenly sea.
Do not take that scripture bait,
Avoid a boring, endless fate.

–Joe Haan

*"People are forever changed
by the traumas of their youth."*

SIGMUND FREUD

*"Anything easily obtained is
lightly regarded."*

BENJAMIN FRANKLIN 1706-1790.
*Writer, scientist, inventor, statesman, diplomat, printer,
publisher, political philosopher.*

THE TRAUMA OF PRIVATE JOE HAAN

Pain was the overriding emotion that dominated Joe's entire being.

Joe struggled with the contrast between the bleakness of *"survival of the fittest"* and the unlimited scope and depth of the human heart.

He knew and felt both extremes.

I was spawned of the Tree of Life,
Ate the fruit with little strife,
I knew not then who I were—
(With so simple of mind, I did not care).
I roamed the forest, roamed the plain,
Knew not whence, or where I came.
As time passed by, I stood upright,
Learned to hunt, to kill, and to fight.
–Joe Haan

> *"Suffering makes men think, Thinking makes men wise, And wise men know The path to salvation is hard."*
>
> —JOE HAAN

Veterans in Crisis

TO BE EMPOWERED, THE DOC SAYS…

"THE PATH TO SALVATION IS AS NARROW, AND AS DIFFICULT TO WALK AS A RAZOR'S EDGE."

W. SOMERSET MAUGHAM

"THE RAZOR'S EDGE"

THE STORY OF A MAN WHO FOUND A FAITH

A NOVEL BY W. SOMERSET MAUGHAM

JOE WOULD OFTEN SAY:

"THE PATH TO SALVATION IS DIFFICULT TO CROSS OVER,

LIKE THE SHARP EDGE OF THE RAZOR, SO SAY THE WISE."

GROWING UP POOR IN ST. PAUL, MINNESOTA

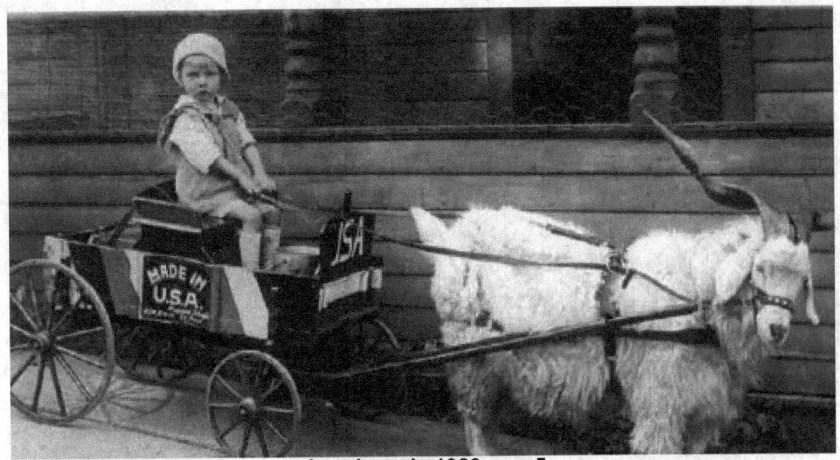

Joe above in 1923, age 5

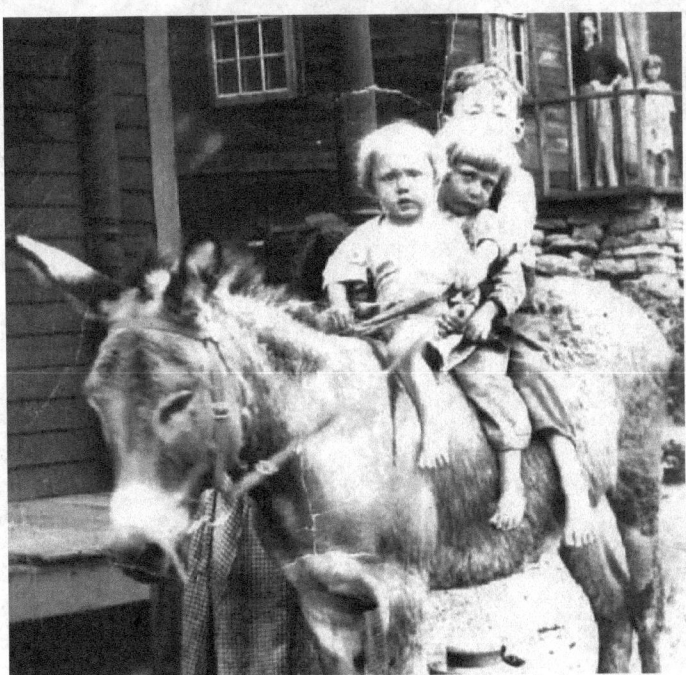

Joe's sister Bub and brother Kenny sit behind Joe in front; their mother and Joe's older sister, Sis are on the porch by their home at 554 Rice Street in St. Paul, Minnesota, 1921.

Veterans in Crisis

TO BE EMPOWERED, THE DOC SAYS...

"ONLY THE DEAD HAVE SEEN THE END OF WAR."
GEORGE SANTAYANA

Joe's Story

Joe was seven when his mother died at the age of 45 in September 1925. It tore the heart out of him—searing and branding him, pain he felt his entire life.

Stunted by poor diet, frequently facing what he later learned were the numbing pangs of constant hunger, Joe wrote *"The Vagabond Road."*

Joe's poem speaks of the bitter agony of a seven year-old boy's "Small Frail Hands on a Coffin Gray," an agony that remained throughout his life.

"DEATH OF A SAINTED MOTHER"

Oblivion —Joe Haan
Time had no womb to enter in,
For eternal time has always been,
Count the tides and count the suns,
Count lives of men whose course
has run.
Organic things within the sea,
Do they dream of things to be?
Ferocious sharks go gliding by,
Little fishes then will die.

Men rush madly to their chore,
To a job they abhor.
The sands of time erode away,
The value of their task today.
Like little fishes in the pond,
They too, dream of things beyond.
When all your atoms have finally fled,
Then you have found an eternal bed.

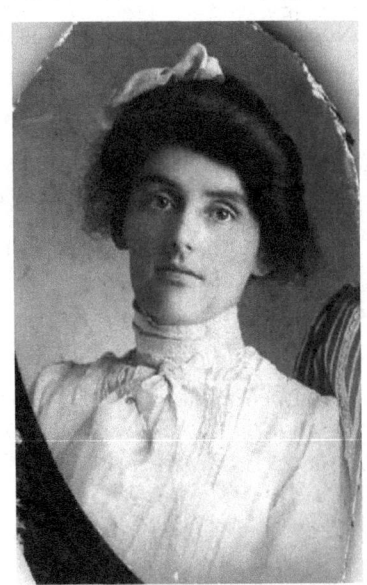

Joe was orphaned when his mother died at age 46

"THE MERMAID"

At ebb tide in a small lagoon,
A mermaid frolics under tropical moon.
Her head is covered with silver hair,
An iridescent body, scaled so fair.
Shoreline sands, laid down in time,
Organically fertile from ancient slime.
A perfect, rustic, verdant scene,
Varied flowers bloom, for mermaid queen.
Beyond the lagoon, a reef does rise,
A natural groin of nature's disguise.
No shallow water, or peace is there,
For great white shark, has there his lair.
The trusting mermaid, swimming then,
Approached the watery killer's den;
The sea came red with bubbled froth,
A beautiful mermaid, forever lost.
–Joe Haan

"The Mermaid" symbolized Joe's mother and the fragile nature of the human condition.

THERE WERE FIVE HAAN CHILDREN

- **Danny was the oldest,** joined the Army age 16, career soldier, WW II and Korea, retired as Warrant Officer.
- **Kenny worked his way through college,** joined the Army in WW II, Lt. Colonel Army Reserve.
- **Rose ("Sis") was the oldest sister,** took care of Joe after mother died.
- **Cecilia ("Bub"),** attended Catholic School after the Orphanage.
- **Joe ("Honey" or "Little Joe"),** the youngest.

In 1926, Joe and his two older sisters were made wards of the state of Minnesota and consigned to the Owatonna Orphanage, 60 miles south of the Twin Cities.

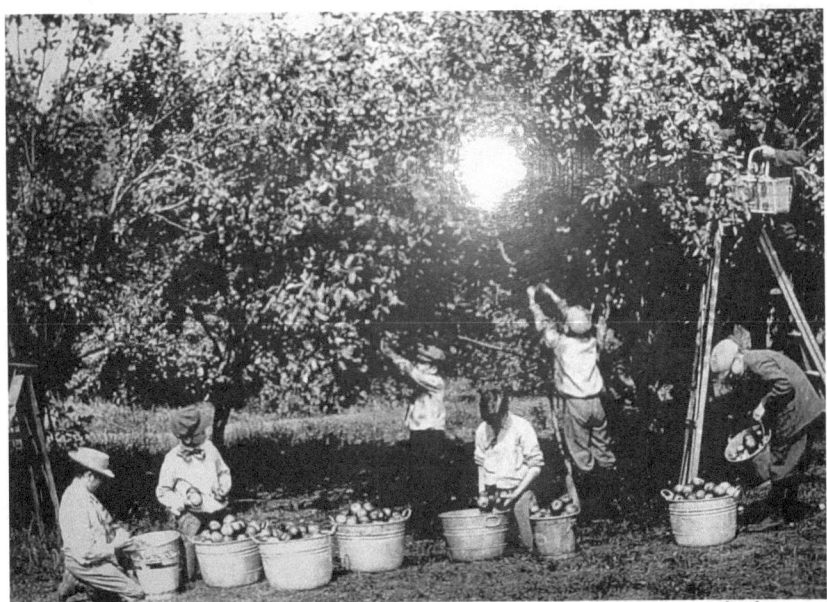

The Owatonna Orphanage was a self-sufficient farm. Everyone worked.

ORPHANED AT THE AGE OF SEVEN

"Small Frail Hands on a Coffin Gray"

In the year of our Lord 1925,
Like any other year,
Many human tragedies occurred,
For certainly the whole pudding of life
Is well-seasoned with such.
So quite early in the morning,
We find an undersized seven-year-old boy,
Clutching the side of a cheap, gray coffin,
Within the confines of a third-rate mortuary,
In the seedy slum of a large Minnesota city.
Streetcars, horse teams, primitive autos
Of all sorts flowed by the door,
In a constant sluggish stream.
All day till late in the evening he stood,
His small frail hands,
Clutched to the edge
Of the cheap gray coffin.

–Joe Haan

Joe's Story

"IF A NATION VALUES ANYTHING MORE THAN FREEDOM, IT WILL LOSE ITS FREEDOM, AND THE IRONY IS THIS—IF IT IS COMFORT OR MONEY THAT IT VALUES, IT WILL LOSE THAT TOO."

W. SOMERSET MAUGHAM

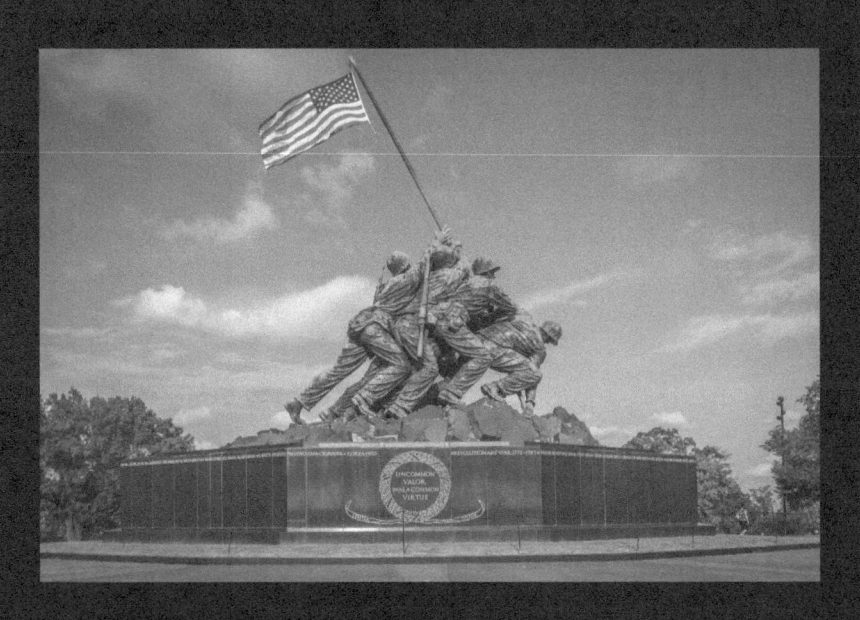

TO BE EMPOWERED, THE DOC SAYS....

OWATONNA ORPHANAGE

On August 7, 1926, the Juvenile Court Order concluded:

"In the Matter of the Neglect of Rose Marie, Cecilia, and Joseph Haan ... proper subjects of the State's guardianship, education, care, and control. It is therefore ordered, adjudged, and decreed that ... they are hereby committed to the State Public School at Owatonna, Minnesota, according to law." -- Grier M. Orr, Judge of the Juvenile Court

The children were mistreated, neglected,
Called "inmates, misfits, outcasts, bad orphans."

https://libguides.mnhs.org/adoption/osps

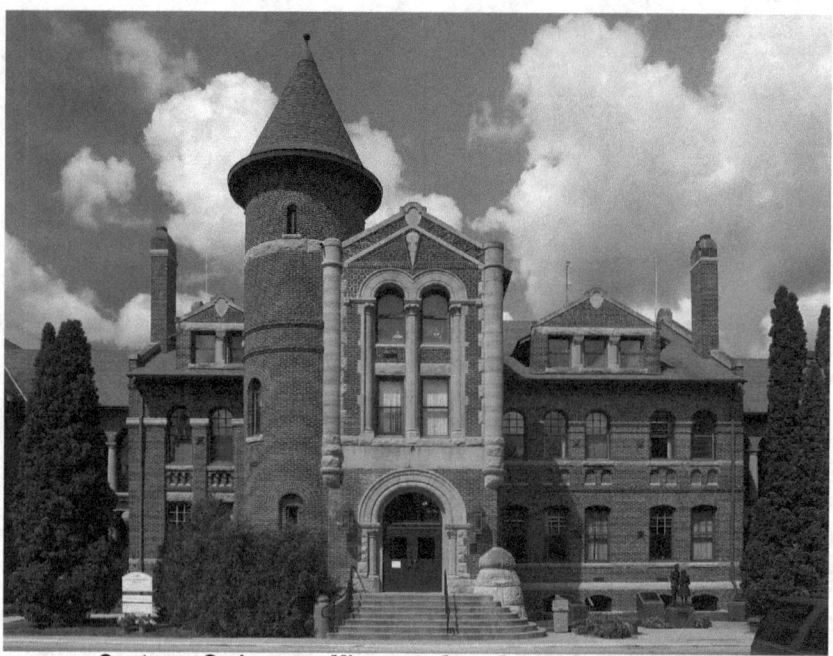

Owatonna Orphanage - Minnesota State School for Dependent & Neglected Children 1886-1945

THE ORPHANAGE

Joe's "Cottage" was *"C-11;"* it had no other name.

"Miss Morgan was the C-11 Matron since it opened in 1923. She remained in that capacity until 1945 . . .

Miss Morgan could be hard and cruel. Only rarely could she be kind and compassionate." —Harvey Ronglien, WW II veteran, institutionalized and raised from infancy through high school in the Owatonna orphanage.

Frequent punishment, radiator brush, rubber hose.

"Discipline, Obedience, Labor"

- The Orphanage was self-sufficient on a 350-acre farm.
- 500 orphans at any one time.
- 16 *"cottages"* (12 for boys, 4 for girls).
- Boys outnumbered girls 3:1.
- Girls generally fared better than boys.
- Frequent punishment.
- Radiator brush, rubber hose.
- Discipline, obedience, labor.

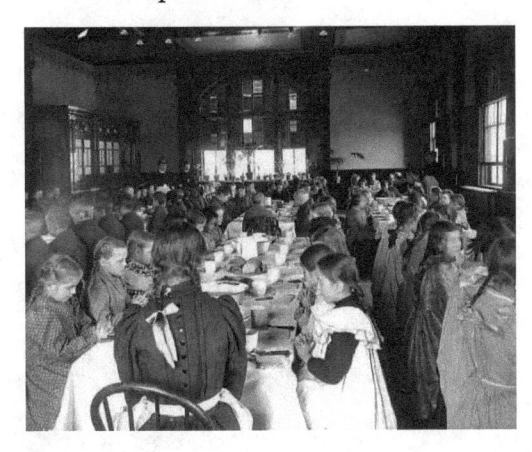

Noon meal at Owatonna Orphanage

Veterans in Crisis

TO BE EMPOWERED, THE DOC SAYS...

"YOUR PAST IS NOT YOUR FUTURE."

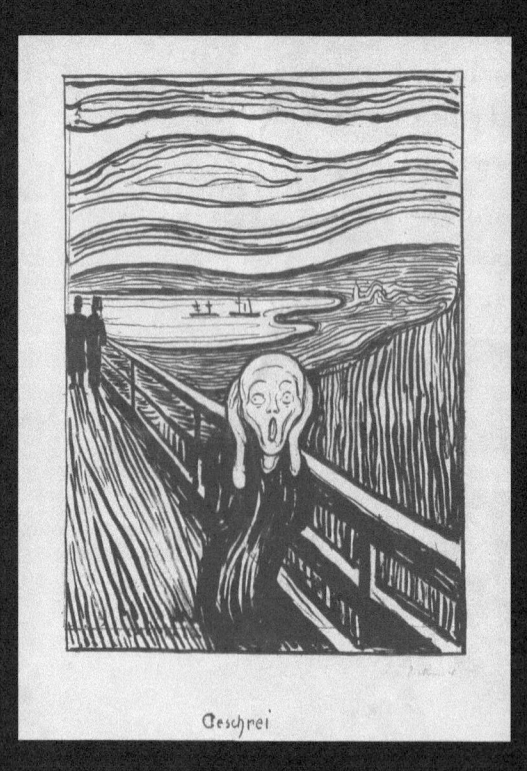

OWATONNA ORPHANAGE

"No crying allowed."

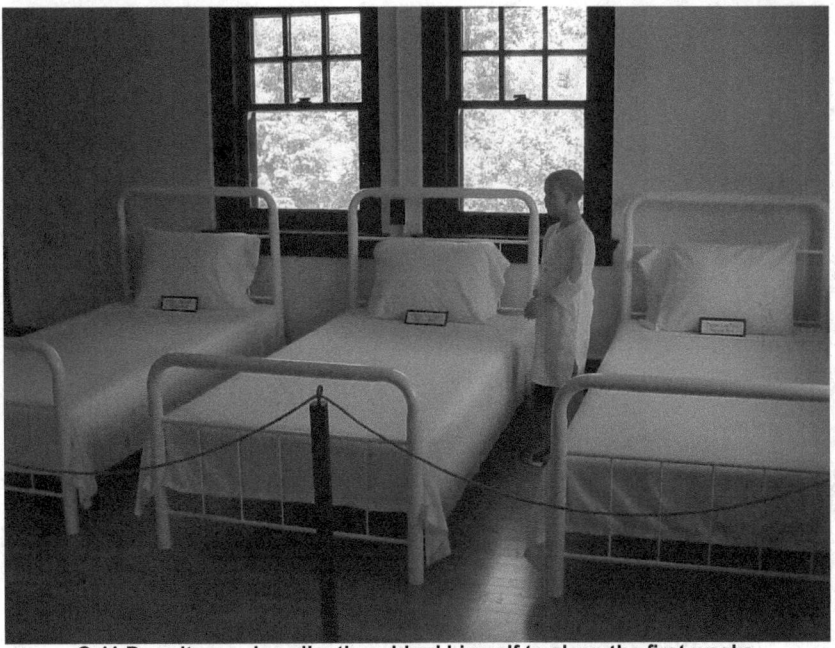

C-11 Dormitory – Joe silently sobbed himself to sleep the first weeks.

"You competed for everything—lose or win, you had to go on."

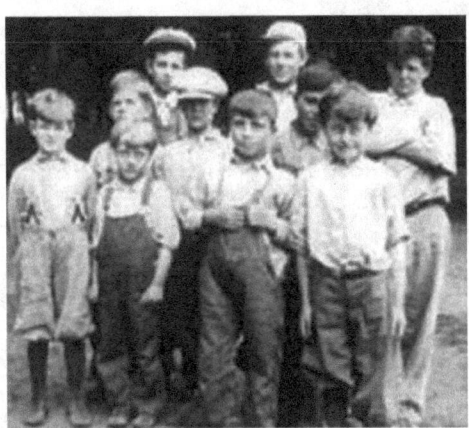

The Boys from C-11.

Veterans in Crisis

TO BE EMPOWERED, THE DOC SAYS...

"NOTHING IS MORE IMPORTANT THAN HUMAN EMPATHY, NOTHING. NOT CAREER, NOT WEALTH, NOT INTELLIGENCE, CERTAINLY NOT STATUS. WE HAVE TO FEEL FOR ONE ANOTHER IF WE'RE GOING TO SURVIVE WITH DIGNITY"

ACTRESS AUDREY HEPBURN 1929-1993

IN 1938 GERMAN NOVELIST THOMAS MANN WROTE THAT THE BIGGEST MISTAKE PEOPLE IN DEMOCRACIES CAN MAKE IS *"SELF-FORGETFULNESS."* **MANN FEARED IT WAS DANGEROUSLY EASY FOR SOCIETIES TO TAKE DEMOCRACY FOR GRANTED, ERASING FROM THE COLLECTIVE MEMORY THE DIFFICULT PROCESS OF CREATING THE INSTITUTIONS UNDERPINNING SELF-GOVERNMENT AND ASSUMING THAT THESE INSTITUTIONS WERE INVULNERABLE.**

OWATONNA ORPHANAGE

The rules were strict. The orphanage was cold, menacing and grim—children were locked in closets, no supper, whipped, paddled.

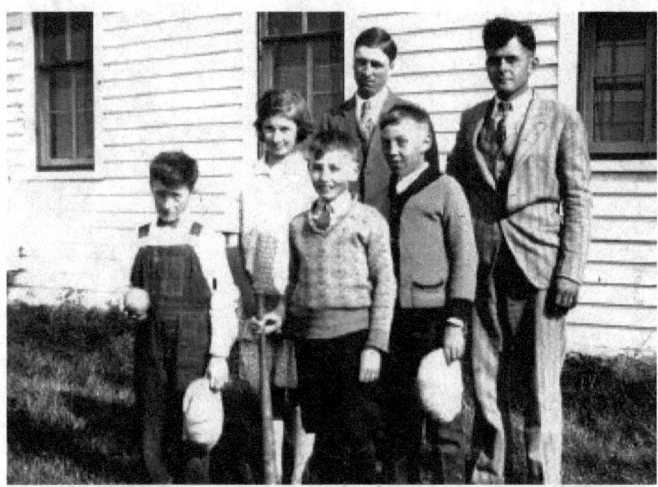

Joe (with bat), posed photo for State inspectors, 1928.

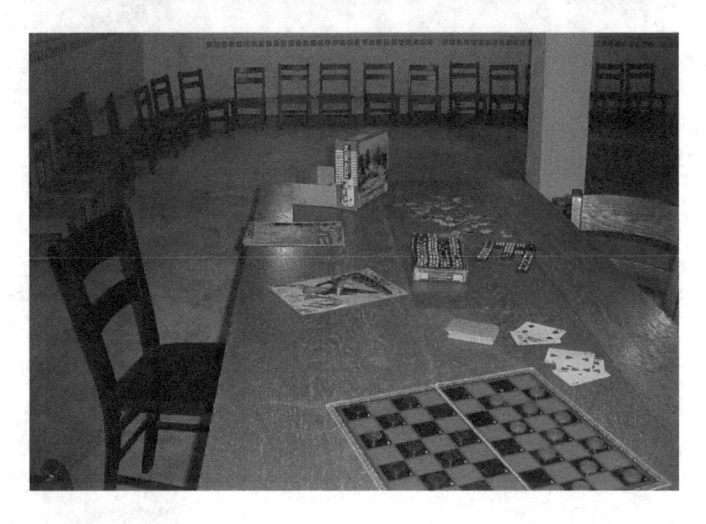

"We practically lived in the basement—each child had his own assigned chair for order and accountability."

--Harvey Ronglien

TO BE EMPOWERED, THE DOC SAYS...

"IF YOU ARE NOT WILLING TO LEARN, NO ONE CAN HELP YOU. IF YOU ARE DETERMINED TO LEARN, NO ONE CAN STOP YOU."

INDENTURED TO A CRUEL FARMER

Under the terms of the formal Indenture Contract with the State of Minnesota, Joe was transferred from the State School Orphanage in Owatonna to the legal custody of a cruel farmer. The farm was about 50 miles southwest of Owatonna near the town of Wells. The farmer was the son of German immigrants, and he turned out to be a stern and insensitive master. Joe was to become a virtual slave; his childhood had ended.

As he looked back as an adult, Joe said life with the German family was like a tale from a bleak and dreary Dickens novel. He lived on a remote, desolate, poverty-stricken farm during the Great Depression, with little food. He was always hungry and worked constantly from sunrise to sunset, seven days a week. The farmer and his wife grew up speaking German, and the first thing they told Joe in gruff German accents was that the farmer's name in the German Bible meant *"god's strong man,"* and in other places it meant *"angel of death."*

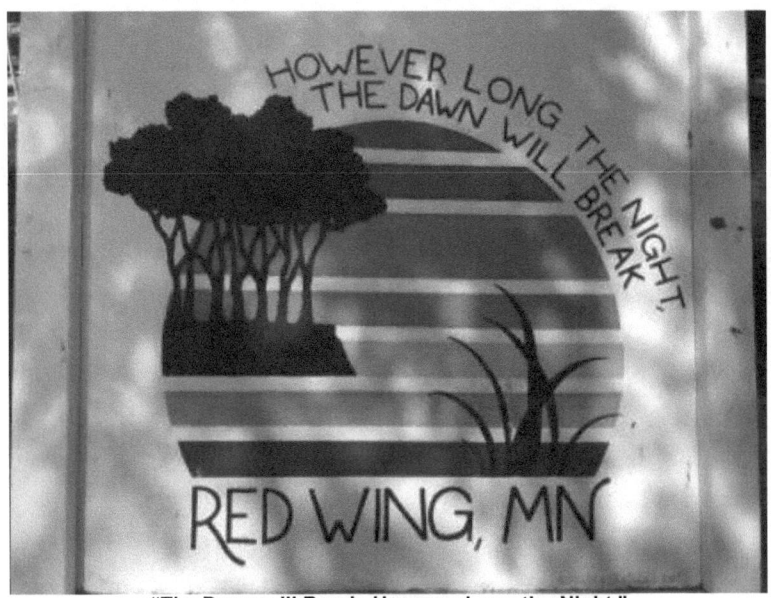

"The Dawn will Break, However Long the Night."

THE FARMHOUSE

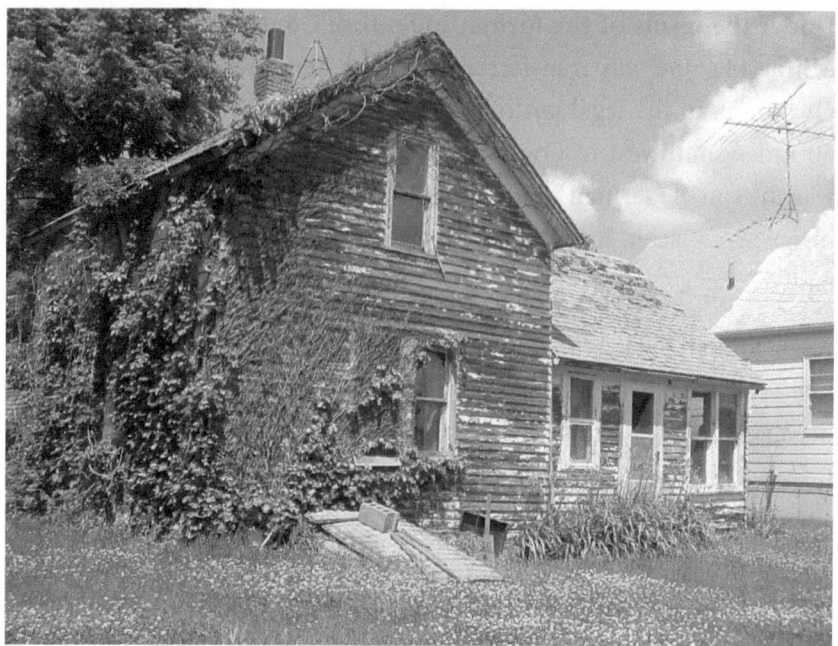

Joe's windowless room in the unfinished upstairs attic in the back of the house, cold in winter, hot in summer.

In the woodshed, the farmer would say to Joe in German:

"You are being punished, orphan boy, for God allows no mockery. The Good Book says you will eat your bread by the sweat of your brow, for dust you are, and to dust you shall return."

TRAUMA IN THE WOODSHED

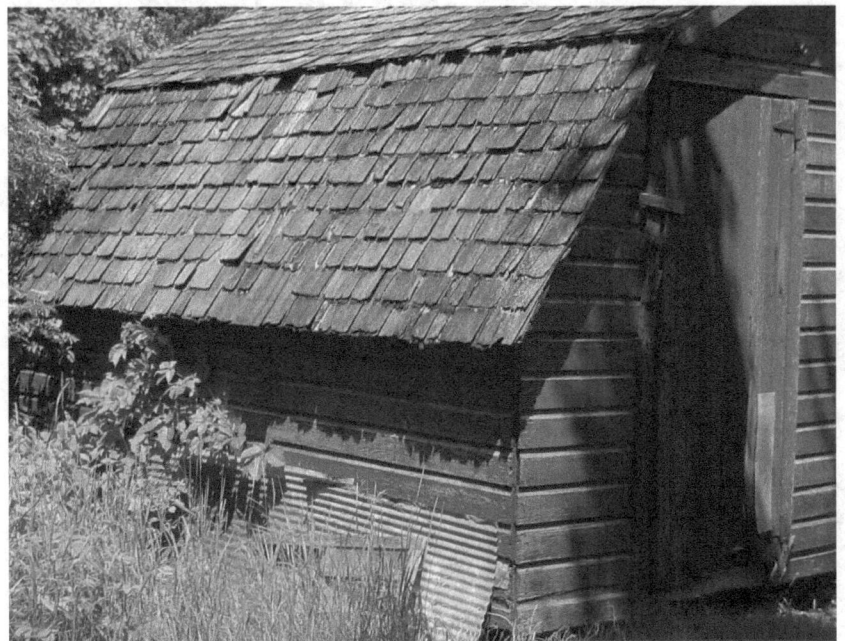

Starting on his first day at the farm, Joe was beaten in the woodshed by the sadistic farmer to whom he was indentured for eight long years.

Joe would cry himself to sleep at night:

> *"Why does god treat small children so horribly?*
> *Why are people so hard on the animals?*
> *Why is god so hard on the people?"*

He began calling himself "God's Angry Man."

Joe's frustration over his bewildering lack of knowledge and inability to do anything about his situation—the utter hopelessness of his condition with no one to turn to or even talk with—made him boil with rage when he came in contact with people. Joe was okay when he was outdoors and all alone, but he was angry all the time when around the family and other people.

Veterans in Crisis

TO BE EMPOWERED, THE DOC SAYS...

BIOLOGY GIVES YOU A BRAIN. LIFE TURNS IT INTO A MIND.

WHEN YOU ARE BRAVE ENOUGH TO EXPLORE THE DARKNESS, THE INFINITE POWER OF A GUIDING LIGHT APPEARS.

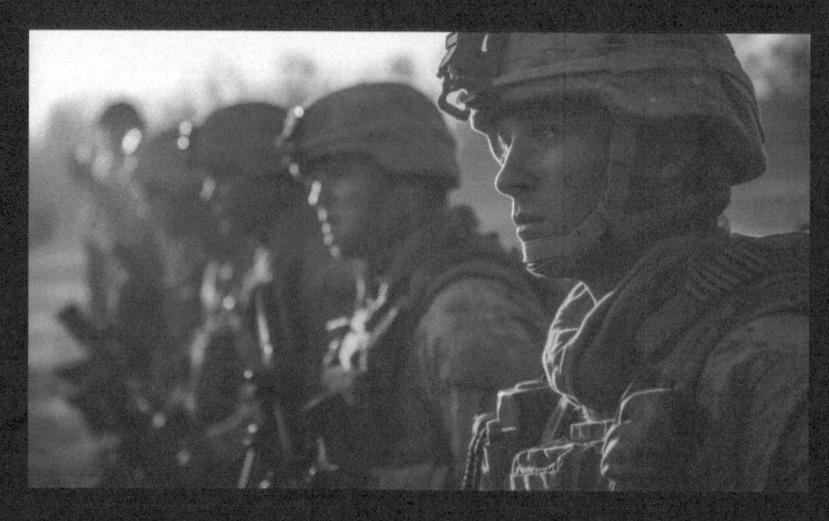

LAST DAY ON THE FARM

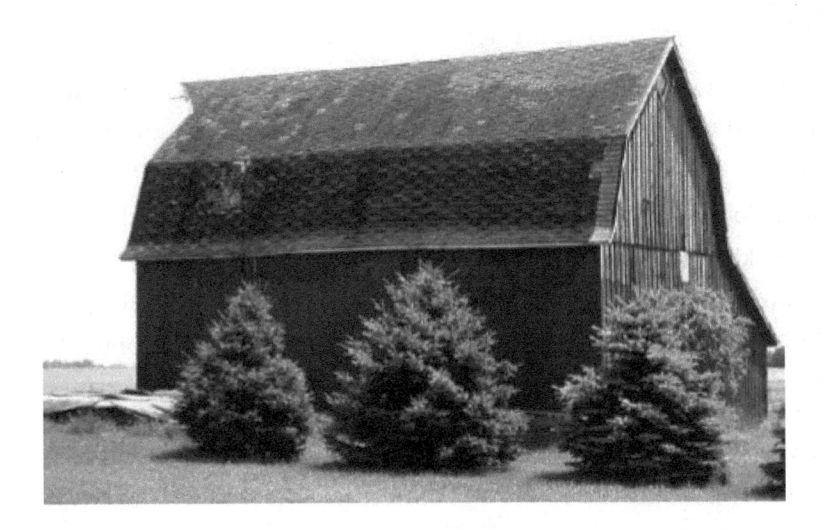

At the height of the Great Depression, more than a quarter million teenagers like Joe were on the road. They illegally hopped freight trains as they crossed the country back and forth, "riding the rails." They hit the road because they wanted adventure, to see the world, escape unhappiness at home. Sometimes destitute fathers had too many mouths to feed, or, as in Joe's case, because there were no jobs and nowhere else to go but the next town. It was an exciting time for an imprisoned and untraveled teenager like Joe, to be set free for the first time in his life, and especially for someone who was so inquisitive but who knew so little of the world except for his observations on the farm.

Joe had been dreaming of escape for nearly a decade. Every night after prayers in the orphanage in Owatonna, the boys in C-11, Joe's cottage, would secretly plot their escapes, as though they were big-time prisoners at the Minnesota State Prison in Stillwater. The nearby train tracks were always the means of escape—beckoning rails that led the way to freedom like the Underground Railroad in Uncle Tom's Cabin and other Civil War stories he had learned from Sis. The boys dreamed of hopping the nearest freight train, and many tried their hand at it, but nearly all attempts were unsuccessful, and they were quickly brought back to Owatonna.

So when Joe had his chance the day he decked the German farmer on the head with a two-by-four, he headed straight for the railroad tracks that ran through the nearest town, about ten miles from the farm. Joe never looked back when he ran away, nor did he care which direction he took to escape from southern Minnesota. Nor did he ever receive the $100 and two suits of clothes he was owed by the Owatonna Orphanage and State of Minnesota under the terms of the Indenture Contract.

Joe slept outdoors and in the barn in the heat of summer. On his last day at the hated farm, Joe hit the German farmer on the head with a 2x4 after a scuffle and ran away to the nearest train junction a few miles away.

Joe crisscrossed the country several times as he rode the rails in the late 1930s. He was aware of the winds of war blowing from Europe and found that by frequenting small-town libraries, he could keep up with the news and often befriend local citizens who would lend him a hand.

He found he could also avoid hobo competition when "bumming" a meal or finding an odd job or two for a few days' room and board. People tended to feel sorry for Joe because he was so small and looked so young.

He liked the free access to books, magazines, and newspapers as well as the kindness, congeniality, and peaceful quiet of public libraries in every community. This is where Joe would go to study, write, memorize favorite passages, and learn from books while he was on the road. That's how it was for an uneducated but inventive young nomad in the late 1930s.

Joe's Story

A MAN SAW A BALL OF GOLD IN THE SKY;
HE CLIMBED FOR IT,
AND EVENTUALLY HE ACHIEVED IT—
IT WAS CLAY.

NOW THIS IS THE STRANGE PART:
WHEN THE MAN WENT TO THE EARTH
AND LOOKED AGAIN,
LO, THERE WAS THE BALL OF GOLD.

NOW THIS IS THE STRANGEST PART:
IT WAS A BALL OF GOLD.
AYE, BY THE HEAVENS,
IT WAS A BALL OF GOLD.

"THE RED BADGE OF COURAGE"
BY STEPHEN CRANE 1871-1900
AMERICAN AUTHOR AND POET

TO BE EMPOWERED, THE DOC SAYS...

DEPTHS OF THE GREAT DEPRESSION

Millions were out of work in the 1930s.

- Unemployment was over 50% in rural areas.
- More than a quarter million teenagers like Joe were on the road.
- No one had any money, especially poor itinerant teenagers.
- But Joe was inventive and learned to survive.
- Librarians befriended him, pointed out good books to read and odd jobs.

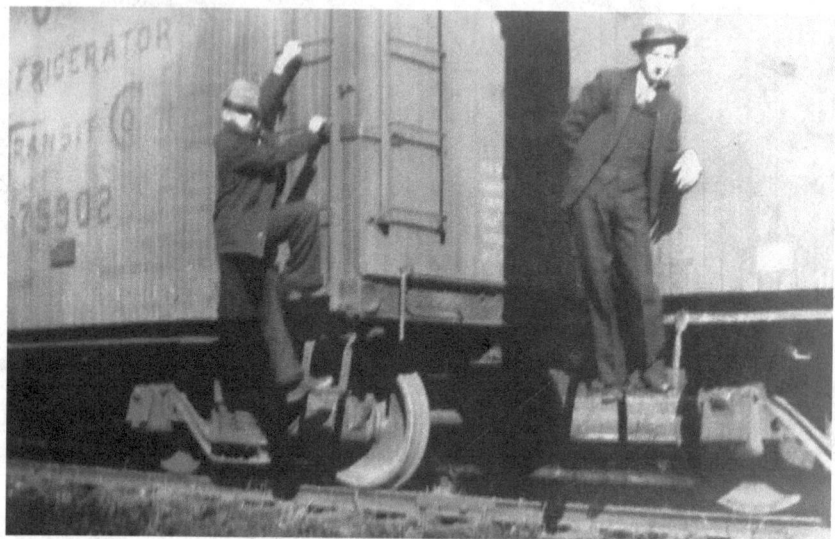

Joe on left, hopping a boxcar, 1937

- **The 1930s were really tough for teenagers *"on the bum"*—** hitch-hiking, hopping freight trains—*"riding the rails."*
- **Joe's hobo years were educational**—also frightening and painful. Railroad detectives were armed with guns and clubs—and they used them.
- **Joe was clubbed more than once by the yard bulls**—he recalled jumping into a box car one day as a bullet hit the wall a foot from his head.

RIDING THE RAILS 1936-1939

Survival of the Fittest

- **The 1930s were hard times for almost all Americans.** For thousands of American teenagers, times were really tough "on the bum"—walking, hitch-hiking, hopping freight trains—riding the rails on the Milwaukee Road, Great Northern, Santa Fe, or Southern. Without money and half starved, Joe learned to survive.
- **Joe and his companions suffered hardship and danger** as they looked for odd jobs that were tough to find. They became inventive out of necessity. Riding the rails became an education about living on little food, dealing with cold nights, rough railroad bulls, panhandling, social banishment, arrest, jail, seeing men killed or injured when hopping on and off moving trains.
- **Joe loved East Coast Civil War battlefields** but stayed away from the Deep South because of its reputation for injustice.
- **San Francisco was delightful**—outdoor lectures about social commentary, causes of the Great Depression, society in general.
- **Joe's favorite topics**: evolution, religion, and survival of the fittest.
- **California also provided** Joe with the opportunity to explore museums and study the remains of prehistoric animals.
- **Fellow hobos & librarians liked him** and took to him—he was entertaining & resourceful. They felt sorry for him—he was small & looked so young. They showed Joe the ropes: how to catch a train and dodge the *"yard bulls"*—and good books.
- **Joe showed them how smart** and self-sufficient he was, growing up alone on the farm, handy with his hands and tools—reciting essays & poetry, how he snared rabbits & squirrels, cooked in a stew with vegetables he found along the countryside.

ROOSEVELT'S CCC PROGRAM

- **The Civilian Conservation Corps** (CCC) put needy young men to work in forestry, soil conservation, drainage, and public parks.
- **Men lived in quasi-military camps** administered by Army and civilian personnel. Camps contained approximately 24 buildings, including barracks, a mess hall, infirmary, educational and recreational facilities, and administrative quarters.
- **Men received food, shelter, medical care,** and $30 per month; they could only keep five dollars for spending money; $25 had to be sent to his sisters, who saved it for him.

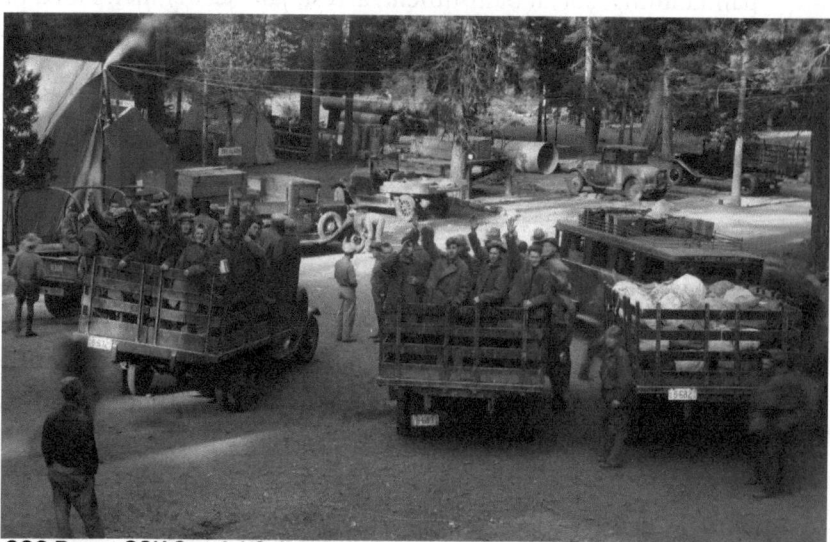

CCC Boys - OSU Special Collections & Archives Research Center in the Commons.
Source Wikipedia

Joe's Story

NO ONE HAD ANY MONEY. IT SEEMED LIKE THE ENTIRE COUNTRY WAS STANDING IN ONE LONG BREADLINE, DESPERATE FOR EVEN THE BAREST ESSENTIALS, LIKE FOOD AND CLOTHING.

"THE GREAT DEPRESSION, LIKE MOST OTHER PERIODS OF SEVERE UNEMPLOYMENT, WAS PRODUCED BY GOVERNMENT MISMANAGEMENT RATHER THAN BY ANY INHERENT INSTABILITY OF THE PRIVATE ECONOMY."

DR. MILTON FRIEDMAN, ECONOMIST

TO BE EMPOWERED, THE DOC SAYS…

CCC CAMP, ISABELLA, MINNESOTA, 1940

Joe enlisted in the Civilian Conservation Corps on January 10, 1940 for three six-month terms. (Photos below in Joe Haan Collection, Schoolhouse Museum, Millersburg, MN)

- **He was assigned to Isabella, Minnesota** in the Superior National Forest in the remote Boundary Waters Area—helped build the road to Ely from Silver Bay.
- **It was called the** *"Superior Roadless Area"* at the time—in 1940 Isabella was as remote and isolated as you could get.

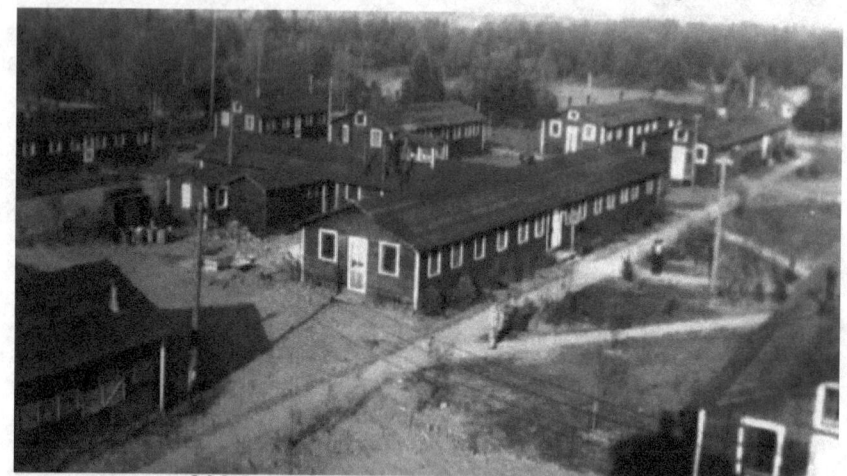

CCC Camp 3703, Isabella, Minnesota about 1940

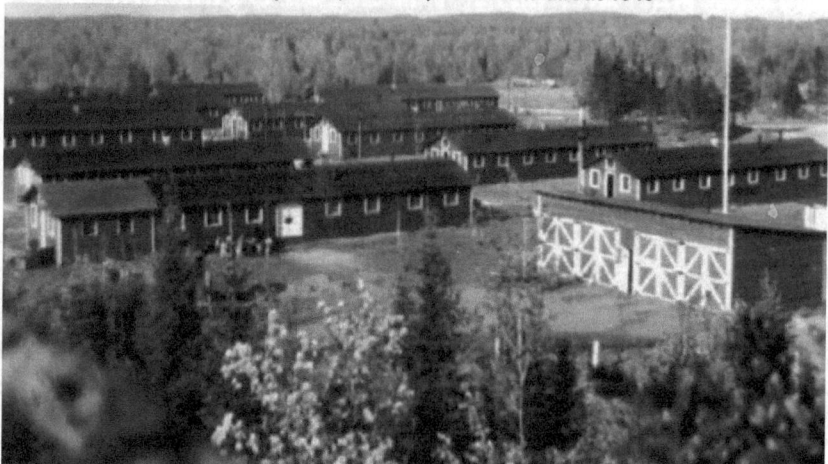

JOE HAAN, 1940, NEAR CANDIAN BORDER

"Lake Superior Roadless Area"

CCC Camp 3703, Isabella, Minnesota

- **Joe fit right in.**
- **He made up for lack of formal education** with library studies—few had any high school or experience beyond odd jobs & farm work.
- **With 8 years on the farm**, plus what he had learned traveling around the country, Joe found that small as he was, 5-6 and 120 lbs, he could handle himself and wield an axe or saw better than most.

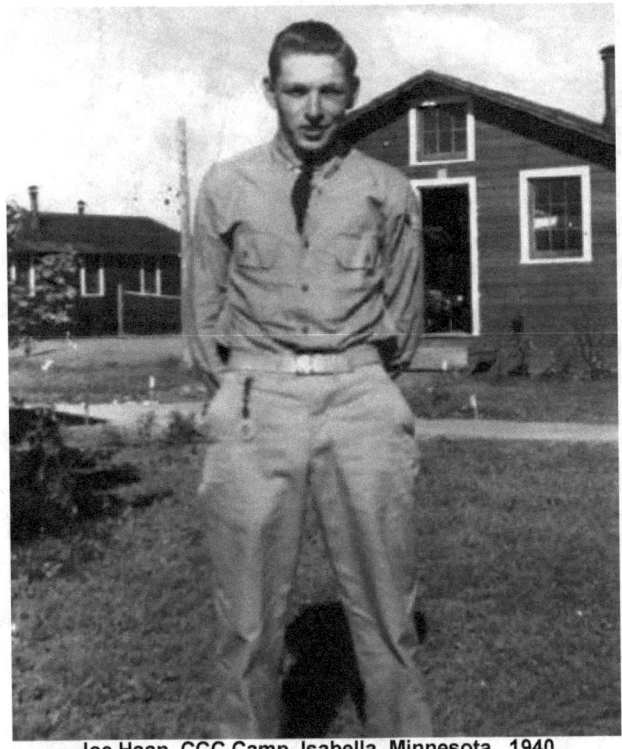

Joe Haan, CCC Camp, Isabella, Minnesota, 1940.

Veterans in Crisis

TO BE EMPOWERED, THE DOC SAYS...

TAKE YOUR TIME –

"MOST PEOPLE RUSH AFTER PLEASURE SO FAST THEY RUSH RIGHT PAST IT."

SOREN KIRKEGAARD

DANISH EXISTENTIALIST PHILOSOPHER 1813-1855

"ULTIMATELY, WE HAVE BUT ONE MORAL DUTY: RECLAIM LARGE AREAS OF PEACE IN OURSELVES."

ETTY HILLESUM 1914-1943

DUTCH WORLD WAR II DIARIST MURDERED BY THE NAZIS AT AUSCHWITZ

JOE'S BUDDIES AT CCC CAMP, 1940

Joe loved the wilderness of the CCC program and its military camaraderie.

- **Joe often pushed the limit** and volunteered for remote work detail where he could work alone all day.
- **Strict military discipline** threatened "dishonorable discharge" for failing to follow rules and orders.

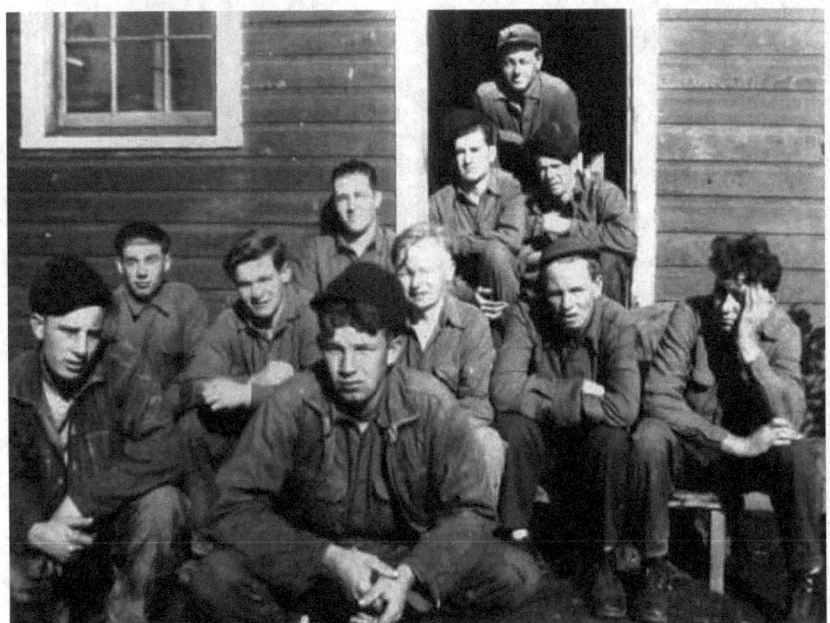

Joe's CCC Camp, Isabella, Minnesota, 1940. Boot camp for World War II.

TO BE EMPOWERED, THE DOC SAYS...

"PASS IT ON."

THE BEST WAY TO PAY BACK KINDNESS IS TO *PASS IT ON.*

"ONE CAN CHOOSE TO GO BACK TOWARD SAFETY OR FORWARD TOWARD GROWTH. GROWTH MUST BE CHOSEN AGAIN AND AGAIN. FEAR MUST BE OVERCOME AGAIN AND AGAIN."

ABRAHAM MASLOW, 1908–1970, AMERICAN PSYCHOLOGIST.

NOTED FOR *"MASLOW'S HIERARCHY OF NEEDS."*

REMOTE WORK DETAIL

Isabella CCC Camp, 1940

Joe said his 18 months in CCC camp were the happiest of his life up to that time; he had his first pair of new shoes, and he was putting $25 a month in the bank each month.

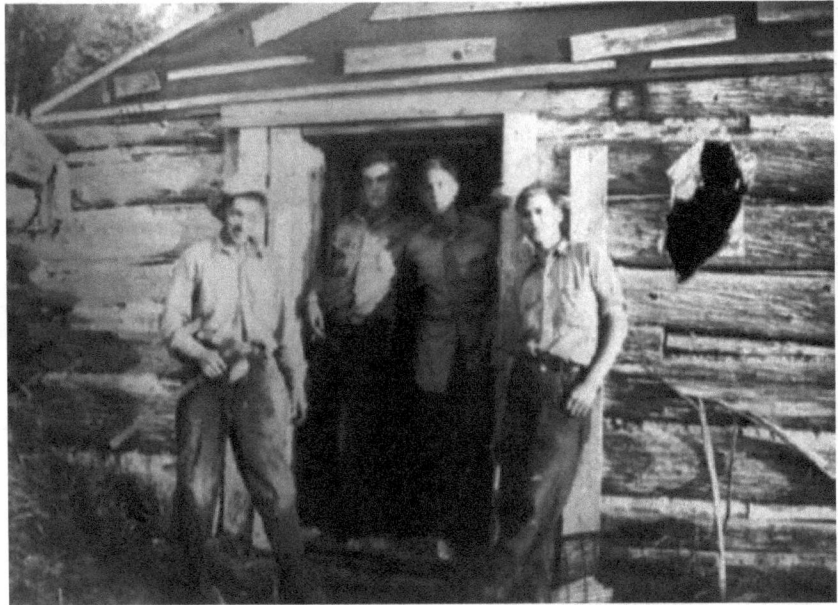

Remote camp, 1940, Joe is on the left, holding the axe.

"The expectations of life depend upon diligence; the mechanic that would perfect his work must first sharpen his tools."

CONFUCIUS
ancient Chinese philosopher

"WHAT HAPPENED TO YOU? CONVERSATIONS ON TRAUMA, RESILIENCE AND HEALING" **BRUCE D. PERRY MD, PHD AND OPRAH WINFREY**

HAVE YOU EVER WONDERED "WHY DID I DO THAT?" OR "WHY CAN'T I JUST CONTROL MY BEHAVIOR?"

OTHERS MAY JUDGE REACTIONS AND THINK, "WHAT'S WRONG WITH THAT PERSON?"

WHEN QUESTIONING OUR EMOTIONS, IT'S EASY TO PLACE THE BLAME ON OURSELVES; HOLDING OURSELVES AND THOSE AROUND US TO AN IMPOSSIBLE STANDARD. IT'S TIME WE STARTED ASKING A DIFFERENT QUESTION.

BRAIN AND TRAUMA EXPERT DR. BRUCE PERRY AND OPRAH WINFREY OFFER A GROUNDBREAKING AND PROFOUND SHIFT FROM ASKING "WHAT'S WRONG WITH YOU?" TO "WHAT HAPPENED TO YOU?"

OPRAH WINFREY SHARES STORIES FROM HER OWN PAST, UNDERSTANDING THROUGH EXPERIENCE THE VULNERABILITY THAT COMES FROM FACING TRAUMA AND ADVERSITY AT A YOUNG AGE.

OPRAH AND DR. PERRY FOCUS ON UNDERSTANDING PEOPLE, BEHAVIOR, AND OURSELVES. IT'S A SUBTLE BUT PROFOUND SHIFT IN THE APPROACH TO TRAUMA THAT ALLOWS US TO UNDERSTAND OUR PASTS IN ORDER TO CLEAR A PATH TO OUR FUTURE— OPENING THE DOOR TO RESILIENCE AND HEALING IN A PROVEN, POWERFUL WAY.

CCC CAMP 1941

Joe learned to play the guitar riding the rails around the country from 1936-1940 & in CCC camp.

- **Joe played his guitar and harmonica in the evening**, listened to stories and told his own, composed poems and sad love songs for everyone's amusement.
- **And a variety of books and magazines** were available in the library.

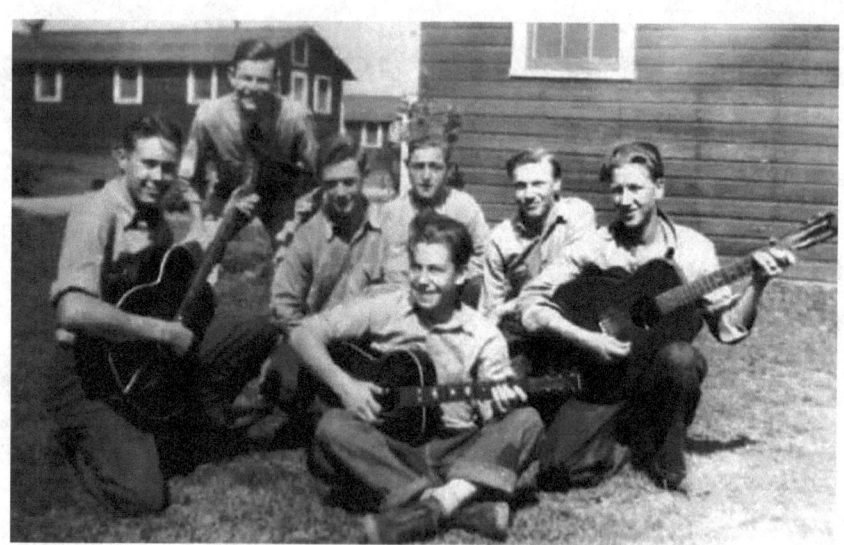

CCC Camp 3703, Isabella, Minnesota 1940.

END OF CCC CAMP

- **Joe received his Honorable Discharge** from the CCC program on June 25, 1941.
- **He fished & hunted all summer** and fall along the Canadian border.
- **He returned to St. Paul for Thanksgiving**—his older sisters were now married and had started their families.
- **The Japanese attack on Pearl Harbor** was Sunday, December 7, 1941—*"a date which will live in infamy."*
- **By the time the CCC program ended**, the nation was entering World War II—more than 2.5 million men had served in more than 4,500 camps across the country.
- **The men had planted over 3 billion trees**, fought soil erosion and forest fires, and occasionally dealt with natural disasters such as hurricanes, floods, and droughts.

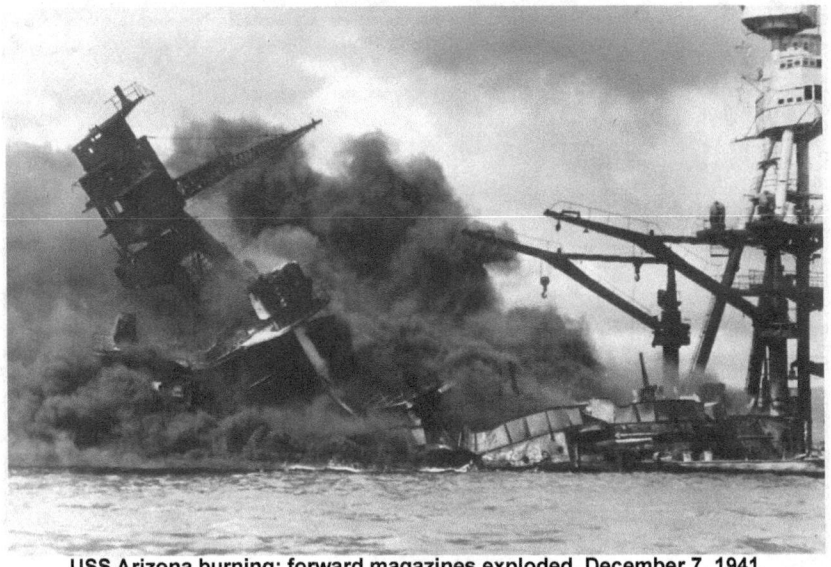

USS Arizona burning; forward magazines exploded, December 7, 1941.

"WHEN WE GO TO WAR, MORALITY, RELIGION, AND IDEOLOGY OFTEN TAKE THE BLAME. BUT THE OPPOSITE IS TRUE: RATHER THAN DRIVING VIOLENCE, THESE THINGS HELP REDUCE IT. WHILE WE RESORT TO IDEAS AND VALUES TO JUSTIFY OR INTERPRET WARFARE, SOMETHING ELSE IS REALLY PROPELLING US TOWARD CONFLICT: OUR SUBCONSCIOUS DESIRES, SHAPED BY MILLIONS OF YEARS OF EVOLUTION."
MIKE MARTIN, "WHY WE FIGHT"

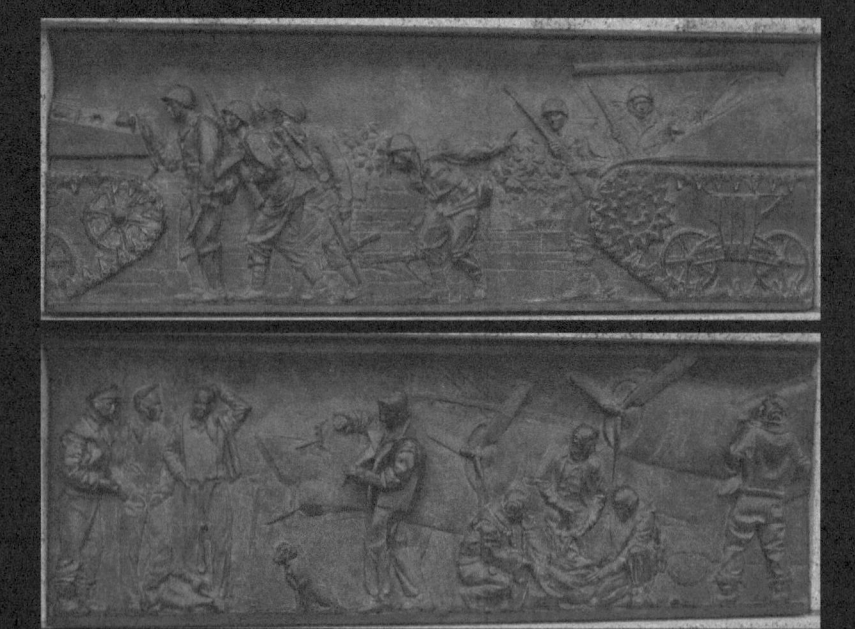

TO BE EMPOWERED, THE DOC SAYS...

A WORLD AT WAR

Honolulu Star-Bulletin December 7, 1941.

Veterans in Crisis

"A DATE WHICH WILL LIVE IN INFAMY."

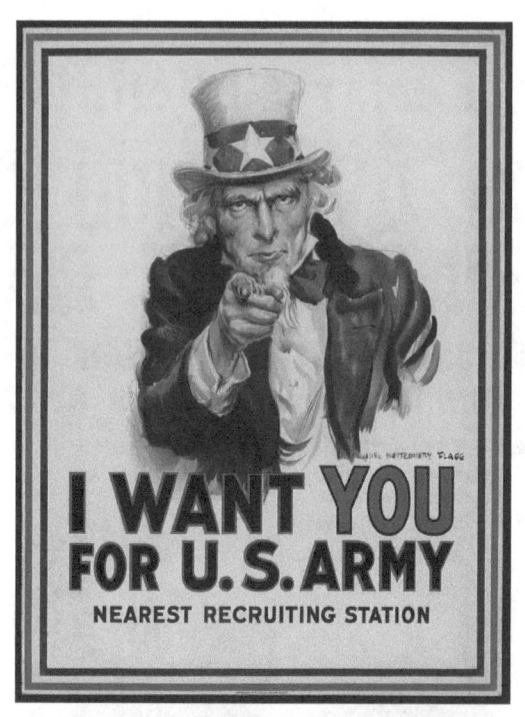

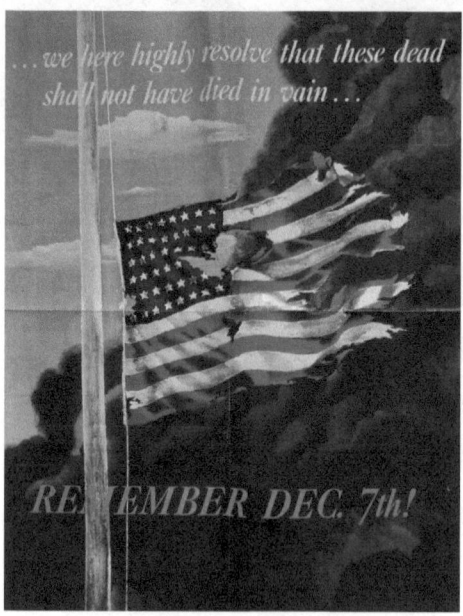

Remember December 7, 1942

PFC JOE HAAN – SPRING 1942

Joe enlisted at Fort Snelling right after Pearl Harbor. He loved to draw and created this cartoon of a proud, stepping-out soldier named Pfc Haan.

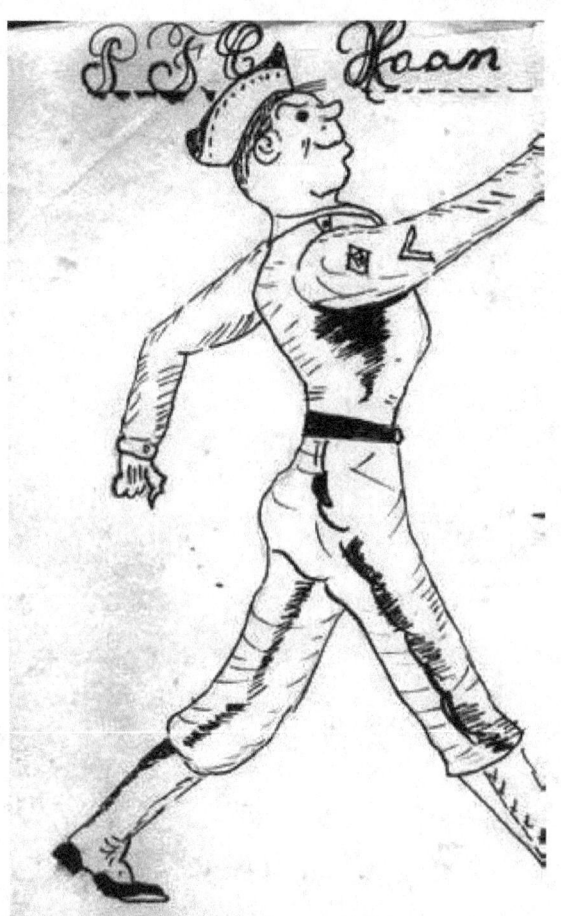

Joe Haan Cartoon 1942

"Why wait to be drafted!
Someone needs to fight;
What if everyone stayed home?
What kind of a country would that be?"

Veterans in Crisis

TO BE EMPOWERED, THE DOC SAYS...

MILITARY SERVICE IS PUBLIC SERVICE IN ITS HIGHEST FORM … NO PUBLIC SERVICE IS GREATER, AND NONE DESERVES TO BE RECOGNIZED AS MUCH.

THE CALLING OF THE MILITARY PROFESSION IS NOT LIKE THAT OF ANY OTHER … NEITHER THE SCIENTIST, NOR THE TEACHER, NOR THE PLUMBER, NOR THE CARPENTER, NOR THE LAWYER, NOR ANY OTHER.

MILITARYCONNECTION.COM

UNDERSTANDING PTSD IN VETERANS

THE MENTAL HEALTH EFFECTS OF BEING DEPLOYED IN A WARZONE.

https://militaryconnection.com/blog/understanding-ptsd-in-veterans-the-mental-health-effects-of-being-deployed-in-a-warzone/

Joe wrote poems and songs to ease his tormented state of mind and inner tension, to make sense of things—the insanity of life, the farm, the orphanage, the war, and death.

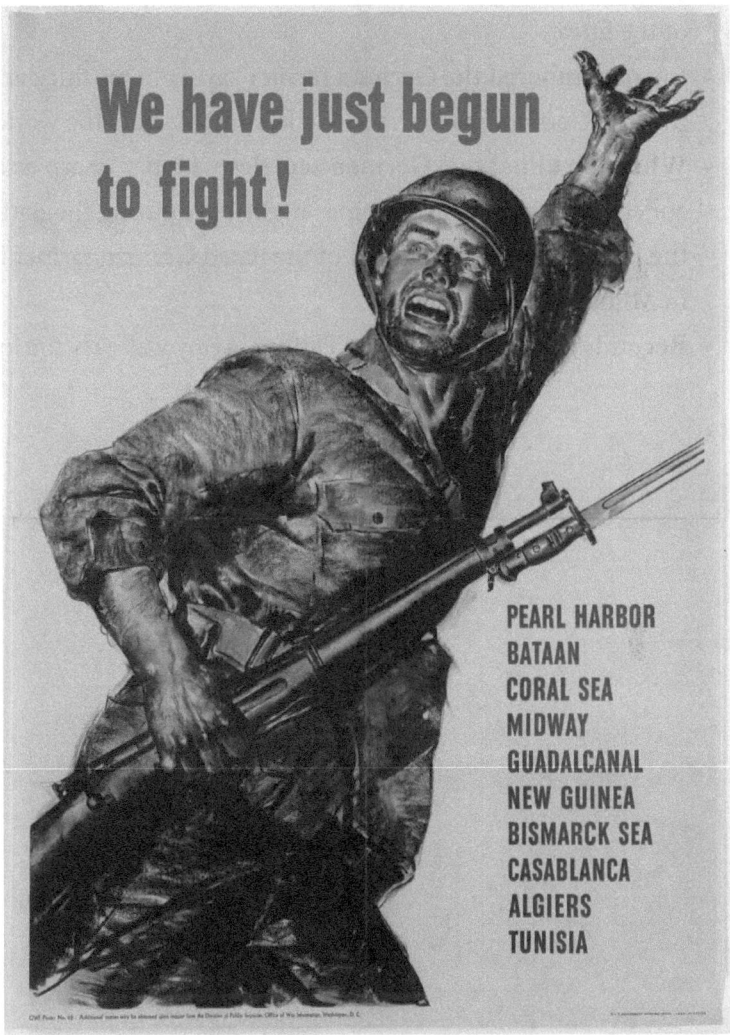

1942 poster in Joe Haan Collection,
Schoolhoiuse Museum, Millersburg., MN

"TALE OF DEATH IS WHAT ONE HEARS"

- **Joe was ready to go to war** with the Germans to show the hated farmer who would survive in the final struggle for the survival of the fittest.
- **Joe remembered the German farmer** saying in his thick accent that the German master race would someday rule the world.
- **When Joe killed two German sentries** with his "sharp as a razor" combat knife on Christmas night 1944 during the Battle of the Bulge; he said he thought of the hated German farmer back in Minnesota.
- **Becoming a trained killer** in Patton's Army was easy for Joe.

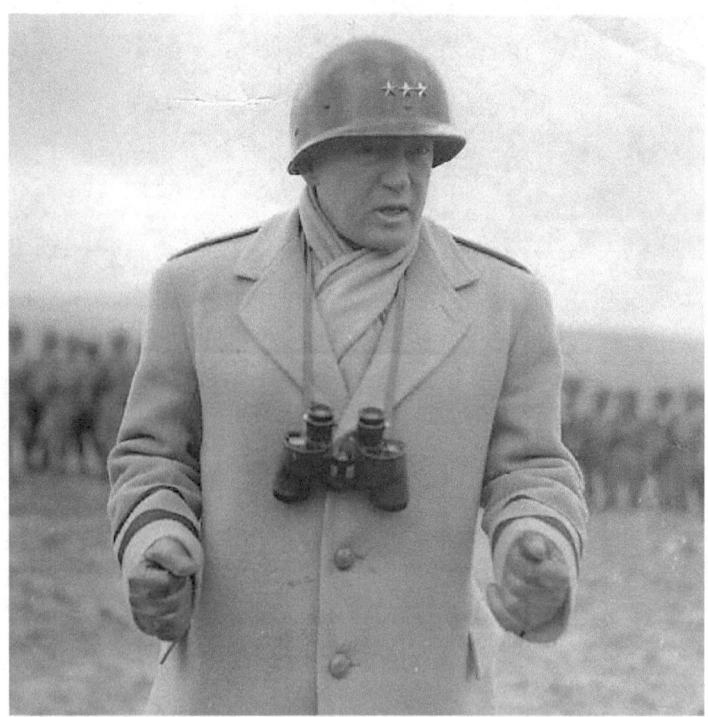

General George Patton speaking to the troops before D-Day 1944

Joe's Story

TO BE EMPOWERED, THE DOC SAYS...

DANGER IS A NORMAL PART OF LIFE—THE BRAIN DETECTS & ORGANIZES RESPONSES TO THREATS USING SENSORY INFO FROM EYES, NOSE, EARS, SKIN.

Veterans in Crisis

"Practicing an art, no matter how well or badly, is a way to make your soul grow, for heaven's sake."

KURT VONNEGUT
American author, POW World War II

"Once the storm is over you won't remember how you made it through, how you managed to survive. You won't even be sure, in fact, whether the storm is really over. But one thing is certain. When you come out of the storm you won't be the same person who walked in."

HARUKI MURAKAMI
Japanese writer

YANKEE DIVISION – 26TH ID

Joe went to Europe with the 752nd Field Artillery Battalion.

- Joe landed on Utah Beach August 17, 1944.
- Joe was transferred to the 101st Infantry Regiment in December just before the Battle of the Bulge—26th Infantry (Yankee Division).

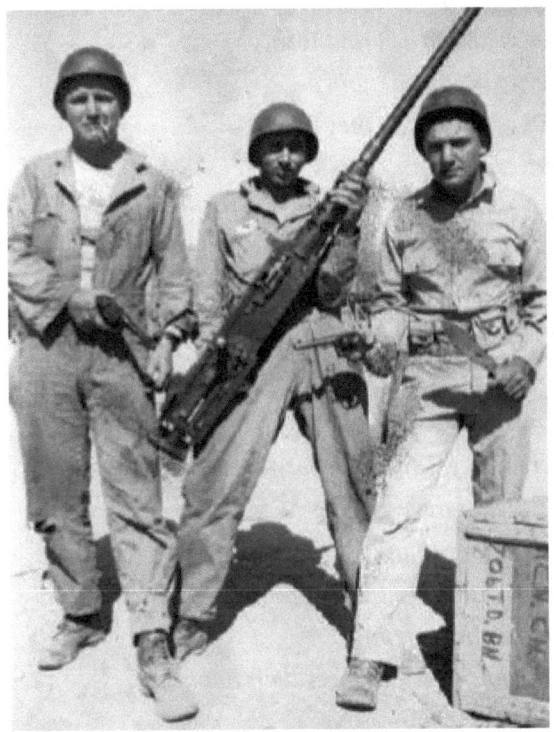

Joe (center) with Army buddies.

Joe adapted to the Army but disliked taking orders. Officers and NCOs who knew him left him alone. They knew he would get the job done and were often afraid of him because of his hair trigger temper that served him well in combat, especially when coupled with his survival skills.

"WRITTEN IN A FOXHOLE – FRANCE 1944"

The world was at war; another formative chapter in the life of *"god's angry man"* was about to unfold.

Man made thunder in my ears,
Tale of death is what one hears.
Lightning flash within my eye,
Giant guns light up the sky.
The earth is gashed, burned and torn,
Fearful soldiers cower and mourn.
So, unmerciful god, now do they pray,
"End this terrible, frightful fray."
All the enemy's prayers, they too,
Have one request for god to do:
"Help us win this holy war,
For infidels knock upon our door."
Oh, sainted mother, for you we die,
No sound minds to ever ask, "Why?"
Tormented screams, from bodies torn,
From warrior men, forever worn.
What was once a forest land,
Are but limbless trunks that now stand.
Putrid odor be death's perfume,
Where human fools come, to meet their doom.

—Joe Haan

Joe's Story

"WE'RE ALL IN THIS TOGETHER."

TO BE EMPOWERED, THE DOC SAYS...

MARGARET MCMILLAN, AUTHOR AND HISTORIAN:

"To call war a crime is to miss its significance. War is also punishment for crime."

WILLIAM MANCHESTER, AMERICAN AUTHOR, US MARINE CORPS, WW II – WRITING ON PTSD MORAL INJURY:

"You know you're going to kill but you don't understand the implications of that, because in a society in which you've lived, murder is the most heinous of crimes ... when you do actually kill someone, the experience, my experience, was one of revulsion and disgust ... I shot him (a Jap sniper) with my .45, and I felt remorse and shame. I can remember whispering foolishly, 'I'm sorry,' and then just throwing up ... I threw up all over myself. It was a betrayal of what I'd been taught as a child."

WILLY & JOE

UP FRONT ... by Mauldin

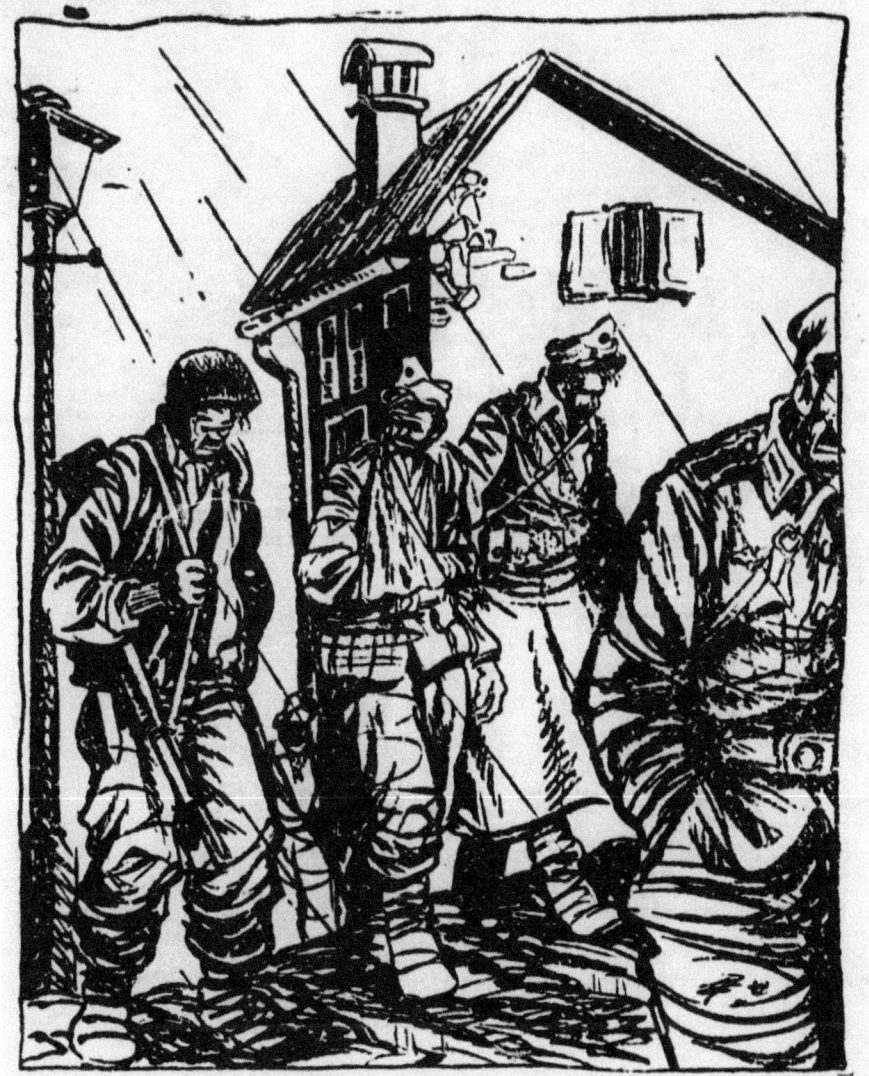

Fresh, spirited American troops flushed with victory, are bringing in thousands of hungry, ragged, battle-weary prisoners.
(News Item)

Veterans in Crisis

YANKEE DIVISION WORLD WAR I

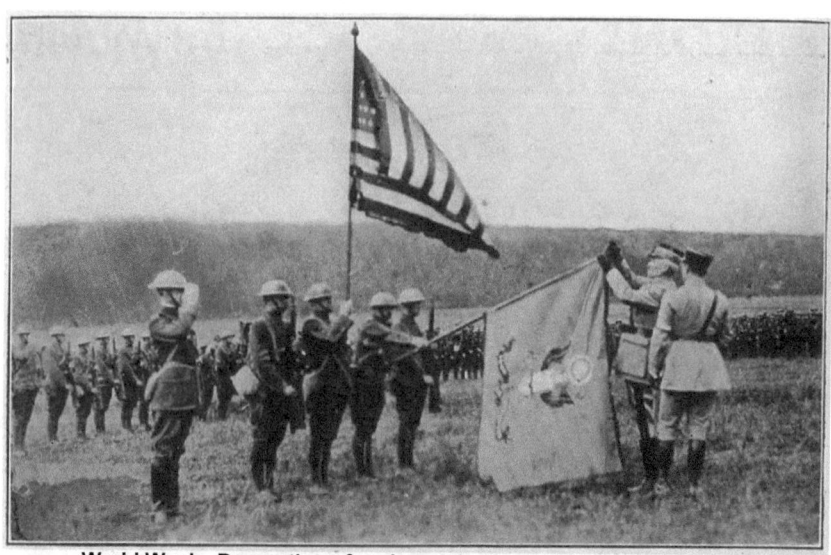

World War I – Decoration of regimental colors, U.S. 104th Regiment, U.S. 26th Division, at Boucq, France, April 28, 1918, first American regiment cited for bravery under fire.

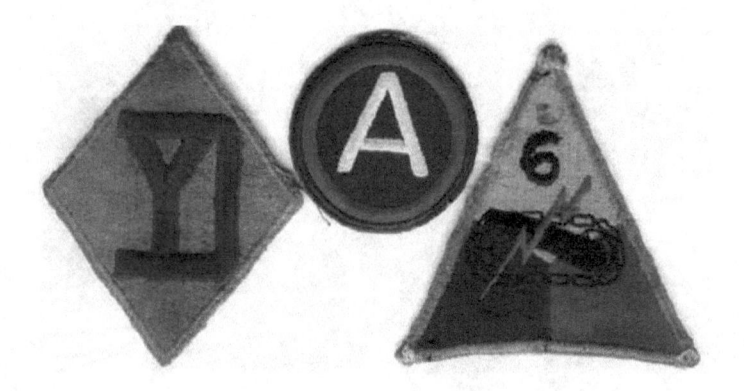

74

COMBAT IS THE ULTIMATE REALITY SOLDIERS FACE

YANKEE DIVISION WORLD WAR II

Total Casualties 16,851

Battle Casualties 9,956

Non-Battle Casualties 6,895

Percent of T/O Strength 119.6%

Killed 1,678

Wounded 7,379

Missing 740

Captured 159

Campaigns

- Northern France
- Ardennes Battle of the Bulge
- Rhineland
- Central Europe

GENERAL PATTON'S ORDERS:

1. Never worry about the enemy; make him worry about you.

2. Attack – Attack – Attack!

3. Never take counsel of your fears.

GENERAL PATTON

"Anyone who says he's never scared in combat is a lyin' son of a bitch."

UTAH BEACH TO TROYES, FRANCE

Joe left Southampton, England, on August 17, 1944.

- **Landed on Utah Beach**, Normandy, France—bivouacked at Saint Mere Eglise—*"piece of cake."*
- **His unit headed south** as conquering heroes—kisses, flowers, cider, and wine from liberated French people.
- **By-passing Paris**, Joe found pictures of German massacres of French civilians.
- **South of Paris, August 28**—saw his first action against retreating German Army.

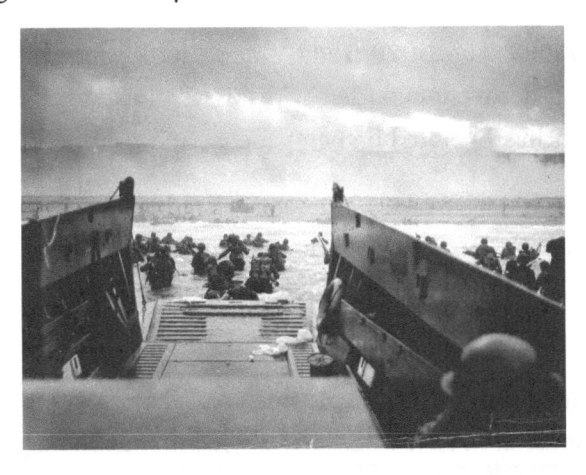

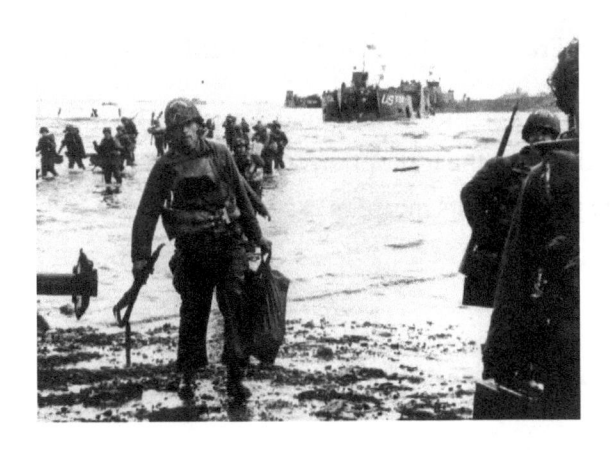

SEPTEMBER, OCTOBER, NOVEMBER 1944

Patton's Third Army was on the extreme right of the Allied forces spearheading eastward toward Germany, freeing northern France and bypassing Paris. Patton used German "blitzkrieg" tactics with high mobility and aggressive shock maneuver.

Utah Beach to Troyes, France

Utah Beach, Normandy France, August 17, 1944—Joe left Southampton, England, on an LCT at 1:00 p.m. August 17, 1944, and landed on Utah Beach on the coast of Normandy, France, at 3:00 p.m. Spent the night in Saint Mere Eglise four miles inland—"piece of cake."

Landivy, France, August 20, 1944—Joe arrived in Landivy, France, as a conquering hero—bombarded with kisses, flowers, cider, and wine from the adoring, liberated French people.

Ormes, France, August 23, 1944—Joe arrived in Ormes (near Orleans, south of Paris) August 23, 1944. Found pictures of German massacres of French civilians. Wheeled vehicles advanced forty miles further to Ladon.

Troyes, France, August 28, 1944—Joe arrived at Troyes, France, south of Paris August 28, 1944, where he saw his first action against the retreating German army.

Near Nancy, France — Old WW I battlefields.

- Digging a foxhole, Joe found a rusting W. W. I German belt buckle with the inscription *"Gott Mit Uns."*
- Joe pondered its meaning...

> *"Under the roots of trees, dead ages*
> *lie down, to cover this false promise on*
> *rusting buckles:*
>
> *Gott Mit Uns."*

- In late October, east of Nancy, Joe spent 3 days trapped in the same foxhole with the corpse of German Corporal Friedrich Hofmann.
- The German Army retreated—Joe's unit captured Sarre-Union and turned back west for Patton's Siege of Metz.

JOE ON GUARD DUTY

Joe volunteered for guard duty as soon as his unit captured their first German soldiers in France. He wanted to hear them talk, see what they looked like. Joe wrote:

"On Guard Duty"

Those that I fight, I do not hate,
Those that I guard, I do not love.
No likely end could bring me less,
Or leave me happier than before.
No law or duty, bade me fight,
No public men or cheering crowds,
A lonely impulse of delight,
Drove to battle without vows.
I balanced all, brought to mind,
A waste of breath, the years behind,
Does not balance, not this life,
Nor this death, this human strife.

(Paraphrased from W. B. Yeats by Joe Haan)

Nancy, France, Sep–Oct–Nov 1944—Joe spent September, October, and most of November 1944 in the vicinity of Nancy, France, on the same ground as the old World War I battlefields twenty-six years earlier. During the first battle of the Moselle River, Joe found a rusting WW I German belt buckle with the inscription "Gott Mit Uns," and In late October, just east of Nancy, Joe spent three days trapped in the same foxhole with the corpse of German Corporal Friedrich Hofmann.

Sarre-Union, France, November 20, 1944—As the German Army retreated further east toward the German border, Joe's unit captured Sarre-Union, France, on November 20, 1944, and then immediately turned back west to help tighten Patton's noose at the Siege of Metz.

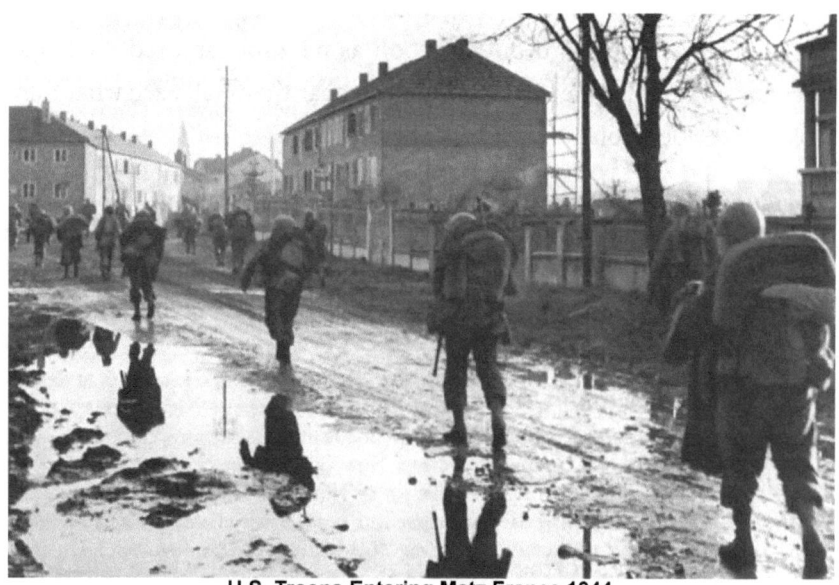

U.S. Troops Entering Metz France 1944

FRIEDRICH HOFMANN

Rank, Corporal (Obergefreiter)
Wehrmacht (German Army—Infantry)
ID # 1885156
Occupation: Mechanic
Born October 29, 1926
Onolzheim, Germany (40 km south of Wurzburg)
Died in a foxhole near Metz, France October 1944, age 18

"I wish I had never met Friedrich Hofmann. Friedrich was a German infantry corporal of the regular Wehrmacht. I met him by chance somewhere in the province of Alsace-Lorraine, France in the month of October 1944."

–Joe Haan

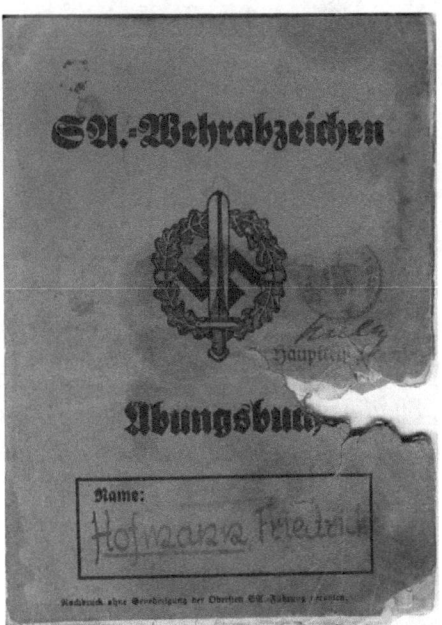

Friedrich Hofmann Identity Papers Torn by American Shrapnel that Killed Him

GERMAN CORPORAL FRIEDRICH HOFMANN (LEFT)

Private Joe Haan, Alsace-Lorraine, France, October 1944, sharing a foxhole for three days with the corpse of Friedrich Hofmann while surrounded and dug in at the front lines, facing death, unable to move in any direction.

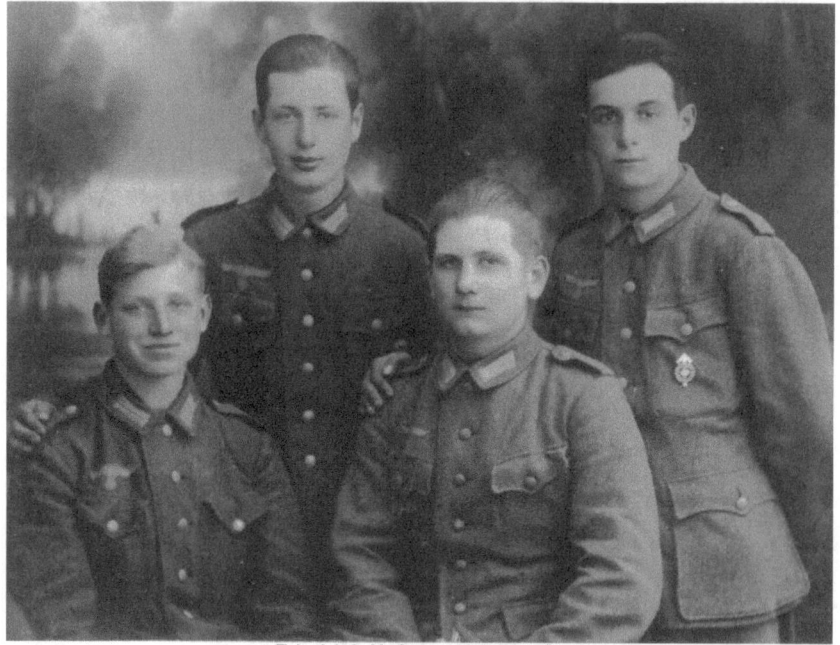

Friedrich Hofmann lower left.

Joe wrote: *"Here I was thousands of miles from home on foreign soil, sharing this hole with a dead man, this creature I had been indoctrinated to hate. Somehow, I had never quite pictured the enemy as totally human. Gradually it became clear to me that here was a victim of circumstance like myself."*

MEMORIES OF DEATH

Alsace-Lorraine, France, November 1944, Joe wrote:

"Resting on the Corpse of Friedrich Hofmann"

A dead man speaks, for the violence that flares about me is shocking and sometimes stifling.
I am carried in a high wind, like the down of a flower, into a fray of which I have no interest.
For all of my energies, physical and mental, are concerned with other pursuits:
Distant galaxies, infinity and time, space and matter, the velocity of light, the significance of a one-celled creature, does an amoeba think?
These thoughts transcend all other events of the moment, while I attempt to keep my poor body dry,
Sitting on the corpse of a dead man, the enemy, who a few days before, was the living,
With hope of a happy future, blue-eyed, blond-headed kinder to love and fondle, a frau to protect and respect, also die for—
"For which I have so young departed, I am the new dead who speaks, fired with nationalism and zeal—
For der Faterland, have I died in vain."
—Joe Haan

'I often wonder why I lived while others died.'

IN A FOXHOLE NOTHING EXISTS

Except the tyranny of the present moment in time.
I find myself completely isolated in my thoughts,
And without communication,
As if I were an alien being in an alien world,
Somewhere out in infinity.
My best friend was blown away,
In a moment of time.
We were standing together, talking,
And in an instant, vaporized by a German 88.
Some men broke under the strain,
Time appeared to stand still,
It seemed that it was all make believe.
Our outposts were about 50 yards
In front of our line of foxholes,
Protecting the outer perimeter of the Battalion.
The Germans were so close to us
We could smell their sweaty uniforms.
Enemy tanks advanced,
We were nearly surrounded.
I thought the jig was finally up this time.
–Joe Haan, somewhere in France, 1944

METZ, FRANCE TO BASTOGNE, BELGIUM

Metz fell to Patton's Army November 18, 1944

- **Joe's division went on R&R** in the city—warm beds, hot meals, showers, first payday in France.
- **Joe discovered French Sauterne** and got in a fight—in the stockade, court-martialed, busted back to Pfc for last time.
- **December 15, 1944** Joe was transferred to 101st Infantry Regiment, 26th ID — Battle of the Bulge started the next day.
- **Patton's Army headed north** into cold, blowing snow—Germans had massed 280,000 men for Hitler's final desperate offensive into the center of the Allied line.
- **Leading as point man**, Joe met the left flank of the attacking German army and shot a wild boar in the Ardennes Forest.
- **For his indiscretion**, Joe was assigned to a dangerous Christmas night patrol behind enemy lines to secure a critical river crossing for Patton's Army.

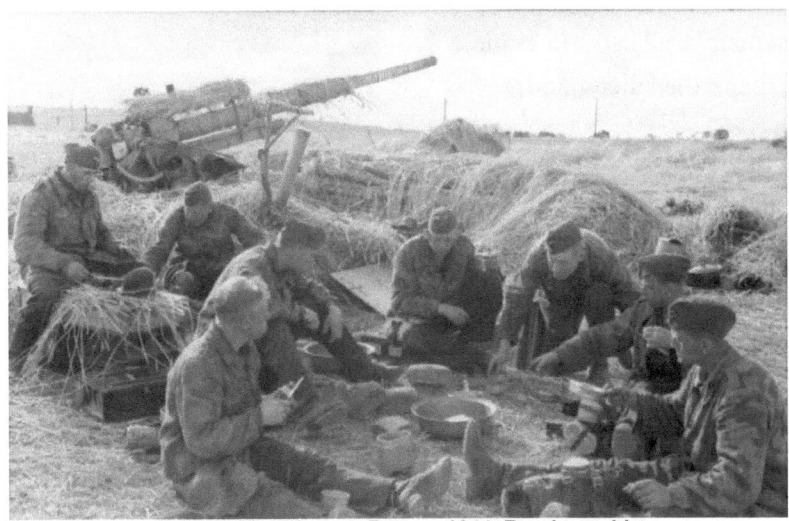

German 88 and crew, France, 1944. Bundesarchiv, Bild 101I-496-3469-24 / Zwirner / CC-BY-SA 3.0 Wikipedia.

ABGEDANKEN EINES SOLDATEN

(A German Soldier's Evening Thoughts)

Speak not so much!
Our last, hidden destination,
Our last desire Is still—
We have written with the sound of bees,
Airplanes droning overhead,
Lands cut through and marched across,
We have starved and suffered,
And with nothing forgotten,
From a shrill scream,
Plunging and crashing to earth,
We wish you a pleasant time,
Meeting in a peaceful camp,
When the dark begins to fall
When the dawn begins to break, rest!
Night would like to come,
Night would like to prevail upon us,
Whether we all can still avail,
We thank the fallen hand?

"Well, this is nuts. At least 30 cannon balls have come whistling by. I recognize them by now from their howling. This whole war is for me more of an artillery drill than an infantry fight. If it weren't for that flooded creek down there, there would more than likely be more tanks arriving. But that deters them. I have to walk a bit, or my feet will freeze."

Note found in diary of dead German medic Gerrit Niehaus, Alsace, France, November 1944

Newspaper clipping found by Joe Haan in diary of Gerrit Niehaus, a dead German medic, Alsace, France, 1944. Translated by B. Wayne Quist

BATTLE OF THE BULGE DECEMBER 1944

19,000 American soldiers killed in action, 47,500 wounded, 23,000 missing.

"It was bitterly cold and snowing, constant artillery shelling, continuous combat, hungry, tired, cold, exhausted. Why am I still alive?"

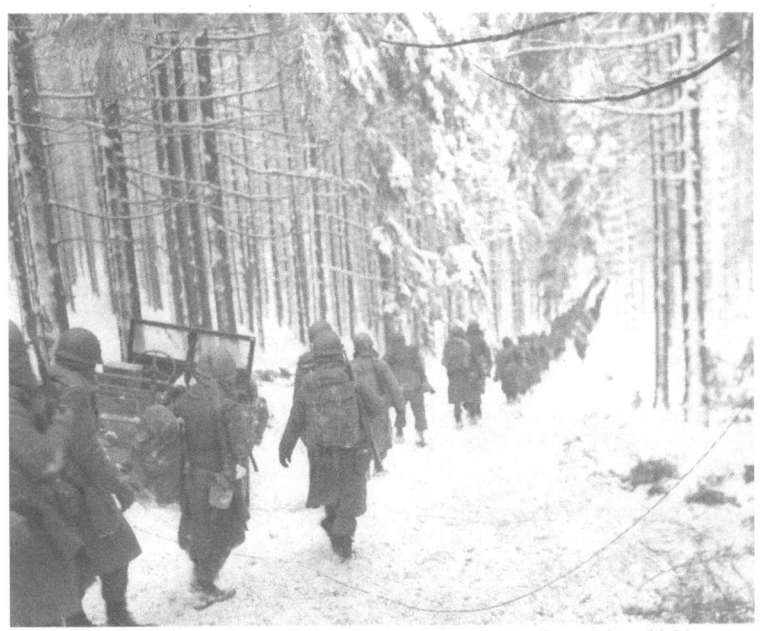

Battle-weary U.S. Soldiers, Battle of the Bulge, December 1944

"Hold your glasses steady boys, For this life, it's a pack of lies—Drink to the dead already, boys, And Hurrah for the next man who dies!"

— JOE'S FAVORITE TOAST: MESS SONG,
AMERICAN LAFAYETTE ESCADRILLE, 1918

For his heroic action 8 miles south of Bastogne, Joe earned the Silver Star & Bronze Star.

BATTLE OF THE BULGE, CHRISTMAS, 1944

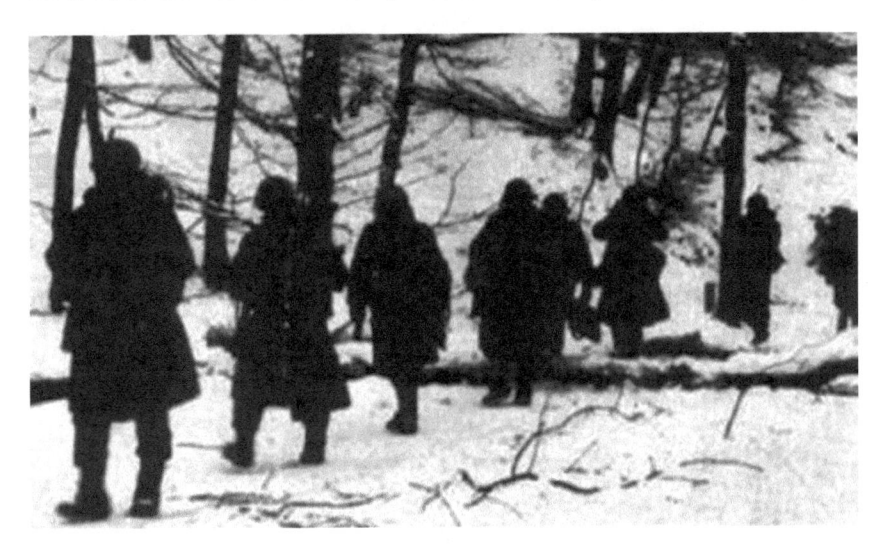

*"A violent thing I do today,
In futile battle men I slay,
Who have been here a year and a day
In time that here they had to stay."*

–Joe Haan 1944

SILVER STAR FOR GALLANTRY IN COMBAT

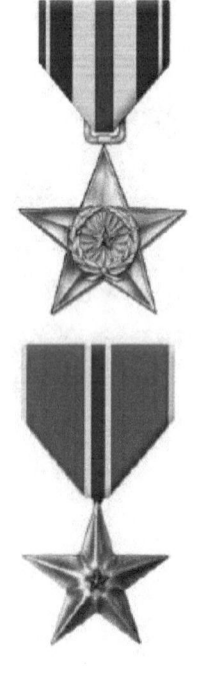

Citation for Award of the Silver Star Medal to

Private First Class Joseph B. Haan, 17047734

101st Infantry Regiment, 26th Infantry Division, ETO.

HEADQUARTERS 26TH INFANTRY DIVISION

28 April 1945

"For heroic achievement in connection with military operations against an armed enemy near Arsdorf, Luxembourg, on 25–26 December 1944. Private First Class Haan's heroic action contributed materially to the success of a major operation in the Battalion's drive into the flank of the enemy's Luxembourg salient. His courage under fire and aggressiveness in action against the enemy reflect the highest credit upon Private First Class Haan and the armed forces of the United States."

By Command of Major General PAUL

THE BATTLE OF THE BULGE RESULTED IN 89,500 AMERICANS KILLED, WOUNDED, AND MISSING.

- **Joe's 101st Infantry Regiment** saw some of the toughest fighting in the vicinity of the Sûre River in late December and January as the German Army retreated.
- **Joe's unit spent February** in defensive positions along the German border and crossed into Germany early March.
- **The Yankee Division** started its final *"Drive to the Rhine"* March 1, 1945, and crossed into Germany March 9, 1945.
- **Joe crossed the Rhine River** at Oppenheim on March 25, 1945, started clearing towns and villages, house-to-house fighting.
- **Hanau was taken** March 28, 1945, after fierce house-to-house fighting.
- **Joe received the Purple Heart** when he killed two fanatical Nazi soldiers and was wounded in action *"fighting hand-to-hand against an armed enemy."*
- **It was a flesh wound** on his left wrist; Joe was treated at the 101st aid station and returned to duty in a few days.

MILITARY ORDER OF THE PURPLE HEART

The Purple Heart is the oldest military decoration still presented to service members. On Aug. 7, 1782, George Washington created the Badge of Military Merit to give to Soldiers for any commendable action. It was only awarded to a few soldiers until it was reinstated as the Purple Heart on Washington's 200th birthday, Feb. 22, 1932.

Purple Heart Day was established in 2014 to honor and recognize those who have been awarded the decoration. **The National Purple Heart Hall of Honor** estimates that **1.8 million Purple Hearts** have been issued since it was re-established in 1932. The color purple represents courage, honor, and bravery.

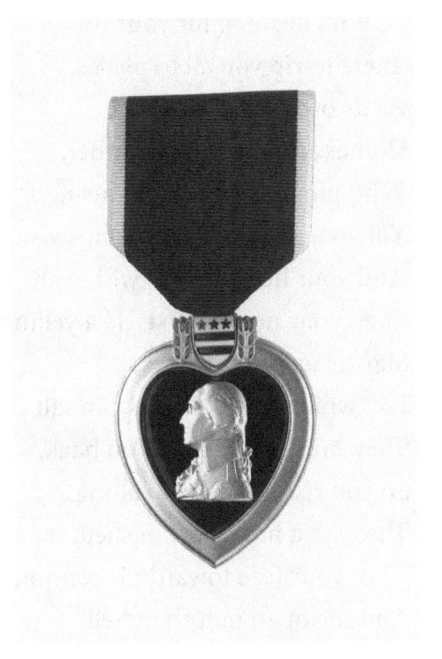

"THE OPEN MOUTH OF HELL"

Like a speeding locomotive
That comes rushing down the track,
You hear Eighty-Eight's a whistling
Just before you hear 'em crack.
And you swear each pack's your number,
That it's heading for your hole,
There to rip you all to pieces
As its own special goal.
Comes another, then another,
Whipping by, or landing near,
Till your mitts are wet from sweating
And your heart is cold with fear.
Then your non-com starts a yelling,
Signals up to the attack,
For, while Eighty-Eights can kill you,
They must never hold you back.
So you rise and get to rolling,
Through a hurricane of shell,
With your face toward his cannon,
And the open mouth of hell.

–JB to Joe Haan 1944

SOLDIER'S LAMENT

A violent thing I do today,
In futile battle, men I slay,
Who have been short years, and a day,
In time that here, they had to stay.
In all our young, infernal ways,
We were drawn to ruthless frays,
Violence, high and glorious,
No man now is envious.
Warriors, we, are in the strife,
To sad, sad music of this life,
As muffled drums are slowly played,
Our total death remains unswayed.
Unexplained forevermore,
A useless passage through the door,
A door that opened premature,
Like many others, gone before.
Grieve not for those who no longer be,
Lost now, in vast eternity,
Return again, oh wretched soul,
To pain and sorrow, and useless toil.

–Joe Haan 1944

Veterans in Crisis

TO BE EMPOWERED, THE DOC SAYS...

"PEOPLE WITH PTSD ARE ON CONSTANT SENSORY OVERLOAD—TO COPE, THEY TRY TO SHUT THEMSELVES DOWN, HYPERFOCUS, TUNNEL VISION, OFTEN USE ALCOHOL & DRUGS TO BLOCK OUT THE WORLD—BUT BY SHUTTING DOWN, THEY FILTER OUT SOURCES OF PLEASURE & JOY."

MERTZIG TO HANAU, GERMANY

Joe's unit spent the month of February 1945 in defensive positions along the German border and crossed into Germany in early March, where Joe was wounded in fierce hand-to-hand fighting as they cleared towns and villages door-to-door.

Oppenheim, Germany, March 25, 1945—Joe crossed the Rhine River at Oppenheim southwest of Frankfurt on March 25, 1945, and started clearing towns and villages in house-to-house fighting.

Hanau, Germany, March 28, 1945—Hanau was finally taken on March 28, 1945, after fierce house-to-house fighting.

"THE PSYCHOLOGY OF WAR"

Comprehending its Mystique and Its Madness
By Lawrence LeShan

"A timely and important book."

- A stunning anatomy of a problem that the greatest thinkers have failed to solve, the question why humans so universally and frequently fight wars.
- Our wars have become more lethal, yet our affinity for war hasn't changed.
- This book explores the roots of war and the practical implications for society and pollical leadership.
- If war can be planned, can we plan peace, too?
- What are the psychological indicators for war, and how can they be used to develop "early warning systems"?
- Are some government structures more prone to war than to peace?

- What are the leadership styles that prevent and diminish conflict?
- When we go to war, our perception of reality of what we are and what is happening in the world around us is quite different from that which we commonly use in peacetime.

FULDA, GERMANY TO MEININGEN, GERMANY

Fulda, Germany, April 1, 1945—Patton's Army broke out of the Main River bridgehead at Fulda, in the direction of Berlin, trapping tens of thousands of Germans soldiers who were forced to surrender.

Meiningen, Germany, April 5, 1945—After capturing Meiningen on April 5, 1945, Patton's Army was ordered to turn sharply southeast and move into Bavaria and Austria.

LINZ, AUSTRIA & GUSEN CONCENTRATION CAMP

Joe's regiment helped capture Linz, Austria on May 4, 1945 & liberate Gusen Concentration Camp.

- **Joe's unit moved from Austria** into Stuben, Czechoslovakia May 7, 1945.
- **General Eisenhower** announced the German Army surrendered.
- **Joe moved to Passau, Germany** in the summer of 1945—waiting reassignment to the Pacific.
- **Joe was in Passau** on August 14, 1945, when General Eisenhower announced World War II had officially ended.

"I found myself envious of a dead comrade. At least he suffered no more physically and mentally. Death can't be that bad; a dead man doesn't complain."

Veterans in Crisis

TO BE EMPOWERED, THE DOC SAYS...

COPING WITH UNTREATED PTSD TAKES ITS TOLL.

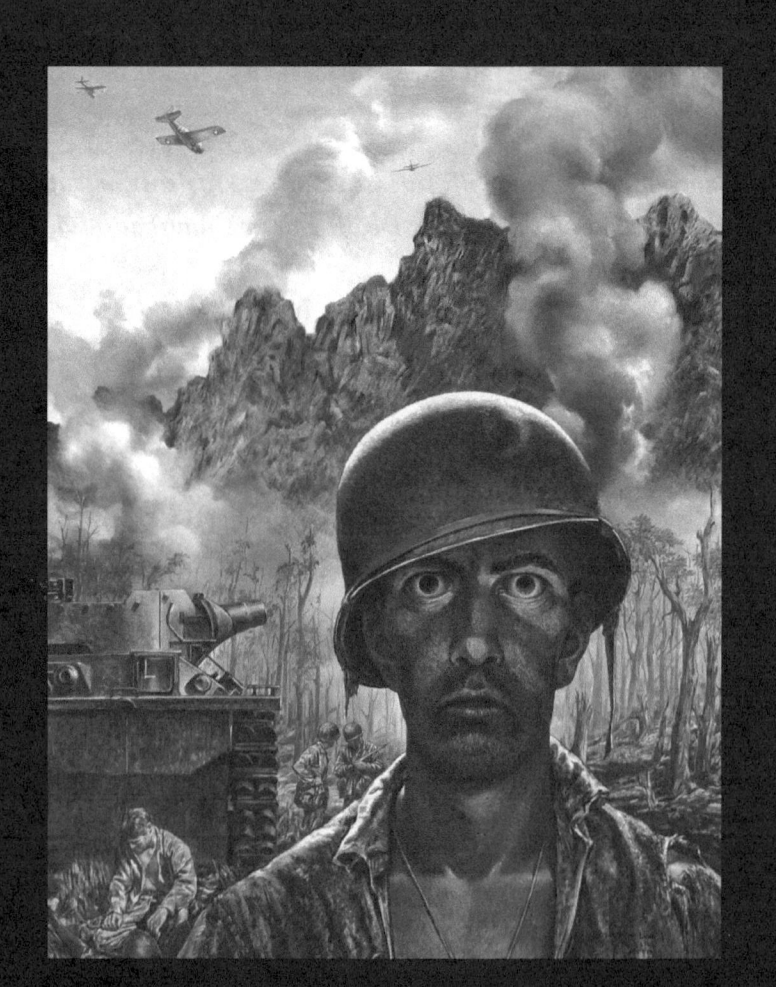

GUSEN CONCENTRATION CAMP

Joe documented German atrocities in a thick album that is housed today in the Millersburg Schoolhouse Museum, Millersburg, Minnesota.

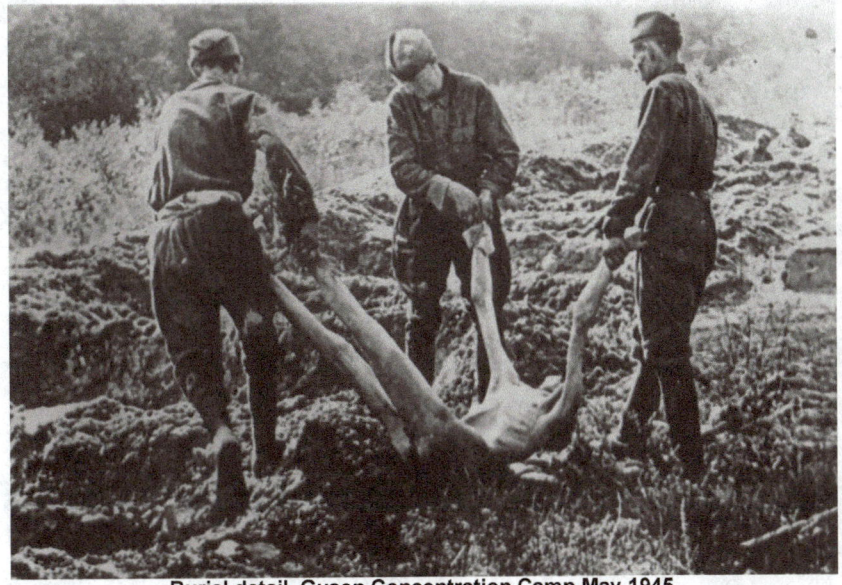

Burial detail, Gusen Concentration Camp May 1945.

" ...if there be a god, may he forever damn the Nazis and their master race."

—JOE HAAN
Gusen Concentration Camp

Veterans in Crisis

TO BE EMPOWERED, THE DOC SAYS…

"JUSTICE WITHOUT FORCE IS A MYTH."

BLAINE PASCAL 1623-1662, FRENCH MATHEMATICIAN & PHILOSOPHER

CHARLES A. BEARD—LESSONS OF HISTORY:

WHOM THE GODS WOULD DESTROY, THEY FIRST MAKE MAD.

THE MILLS OF GOD GRIND SLOWLY, BUT EXCEEDINGLY SMALL.

THE BEE THAT MAKES THE BLOSSOM ROBS THE HONEY.

WHEN THE DARKNESS COMES, THE STARS BEGIN TO SHINE.

Joe wrote several poems during the war, but many did not survive. Like his poem, "War," they reflect a tormented state of mind suffered by a sensitive young man exposed to danger, cold, hunger, and deadly combat for weeks on end.

Beginning with his experiences on the hated Minnesota farm, Joe wrote poetry and songs to ease his inner tension, talk with himself, and make sense of what was going on around him.

Writing about the insanity and futility of war and his life at the orphanage and on the farm was Joe's attempt to figure it all out.

It was Joe's way to cope with his severe PTSD.

Therapist Louis Hoffman wrote: "Can a Poem Be Healing? Writing Poetry Through the Pain."

- Release
- Processing Emotions,
- Awareness and Insight.

"Poetry is often written during times when people are feeling intense emotions. In fact, the emotions often drive the poetry. Much like a good conversation or therapy session, poetry can provide a release ... Poems often emerge in the midst of strong emotions. While part of what the poem does is describe the painful experience vividly and creatively, there is often a component of trying to make sense of the experience through understanding it more fully or through finding meaning in the suffering. When this second component is part of the writing process or the reflections on the poem, it closely parallels therapy."

AFTER THE WAR

There Was No "Decompression Plan" for WW II Vets.

On August 14, 1945, a formal ceasefire order was received from General Eisenhower while Joe and his unit were in Passau, Germany. World War II was officially over. With nearly 17,000 casualties and numerous awards, the 26th Infantry Division was deactivated in Germany with no more worry about going to the Pacific to fight the Japs. That night there was a big celebration but still no word on when they would head or home.

After four months exploring the German countryside, Joe finally departed Europe on October 15, 1945, with a chest full of combat ribbons. He received his Honorable Discharge on November 6, 1945, and separated as a Private First Class (Pfc) at Camp McCoy, Wisconsin with $647.55 mustering out pay. Joe left Camp McCoy and hitched his way to St. Paul—older, wiser, far more mature, still angry. The Army had no *"decompression plan"* for returning combat veterans—they were simply paid off, mustered out, and sent home by the millions to decompress on their own with $20 a month unemployment pay, *"beer money."*

Joe had recurring nightmares when he got back to St. Paul about life on the farm and the night he and his patrol killed the German sentries along the Sûre River in Luxembourg during the Battle of the Bulge. His dreams were about the Christmas night in 1944 when he snapped the neck and slit the throat of a German soldier. A third sentry bawled and shit his pants because he thought Joe would kill him, too. Joe's patrol took him prisoner, even though he got in their way. The captured German soldier was so scared of Joe's violent, broken German that he followed Joe's orders like a robot.

But the bad dreams kept coming back at night, and for the rest of his life Joe would wake up in a sweat deep at night just as the sharp knife silently pierced the German sentry's throat cutting the carotid, and Joe would scream.

Joe never complained or said, "poor me." Joe said he felt lucky to be alive and picked up his life without complaint, as a survivor. After getting drunk several times with Army buddies, Joe stayed with his sisters in Minnesota for several weeks. Then he decided to go to Oklahoma, where he had met Helen Jessie four years earlier during Army training.

Helen was a member of the Choctaw Native American tribe in Oklahoma and had the natural beauty and spiritual calm Joe associated with primeval people of the ancient past. Joe seemed to understand Helen and her family better than anyone in his life, and they accepted Joe and seemed to understand him because Joe was so much like them.

Joe felt that he was born to be a primitive creature who had to teach everything to himself, and that's how he felt when he was with Helen. It's quite possible no other person in the world could have married Joe or put up with him—and vice versa. Joe needed someone who could calmly and stoically accept his sense of pain, massive exuberance, liveliness, energy, and high spirits. For over forty-five years Helen lived up to that call of duty with Joe and their two sons, and beyond.

During his postwar *"decompression,"* Joe would often drink too much. It never took a lot of alcohol to do the trick, and it would frequently cause problems. Joe heard about the ironworking construction boom in Texas, so he and Helen packed up and moved to Houston. Their two sons, Jack and James, were born in 1948 and 1949.

HIGH STEEL

Joe and Helen were married in Oklahoma in 1946.

- **Joe heard about working "high steel"** and the construction boom in Texas from Helen's brothers who were steelworkers.
- **They settled in Houston** where Joe joined Local 84 Ironworker's Union as an apprentice in 1947.

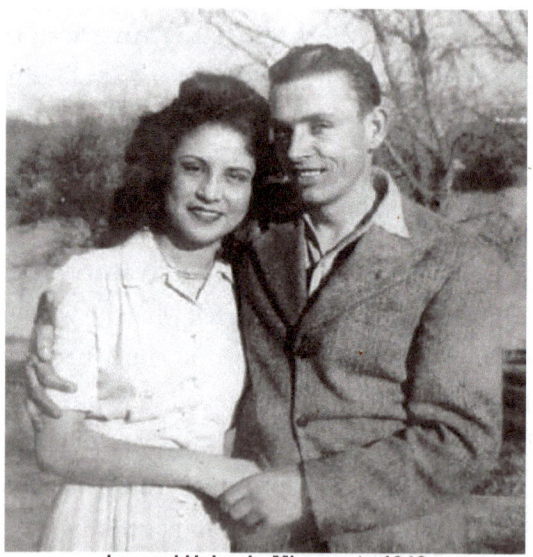

Joe and Helen in Minnesota 1946

Joe was proud he had survived another test of the survival of the fittest. He was free at last—wiser, tougher, more experienced, with a little jingle in his jeans and no attachments to anyone or anything—and then he found Helen again.

Joe received $20 a week GI unemployment (*"beer money"*) for a year with no stipulation on how it was spent; it was called the *"52/20 club."* Joe was trying to figure out what to do with his life, thought about living in Alaska, got bored with civilian life. He hunted and fished, looked for excitement. Becoming a *"high steel"* ironworker appealed to him.

"I can remember Joe having bad dreams and waking up in the middle of the night from the dreams. My parents thought the war had a serious effect on him psychologically, aside from what happened to him on the farm and in the orphanage. When Joe drank alcohol, he was like a wild Indian, capable of damn near anything."

There was no VA treatment, no decompression plan. Joe was paid off by the Army, went home, got married, and found the most dangerous job in the world. At night he would wake up in a cold sweat as he killed the German sentry Christmas Eve.

Joe wrote to his brother, *"I feel as unsettled as the sands of the sea, can't make decisions, if I could make up my mind, I'd be halfway there."*

Veterans in Crisis

TO BE EMPOWERED, THE DOC SAYS…

YOUR EYES AND BRAIN ARE A TEAM

YOUR OPTIC NERVE CONNECTS YOUR EYE TO YOUR BRAIN.

ITS LOCATION NEAR THE CENTER OF YOUR RETINA EFFECTIVELY CREATES A BLIND SPOT NEAR THE CENTER OF YOUR VISUAL FIELD.

YOUR EYES SAMPLE TINY PIECES OF THE WORLD AND THE BRAIN FILLS IN THE REST, CONSTANTLY, ALL THE TIME.

AND YET, YOU DON'T EXPERIENCE THE BLIND SPOT. WHY IS THAT?

IT'S BECAUSE THE BRAIN SAMPLES THE AREA NEAR THE BLIND SPOT AND FILLS IN THE GAP WITH ITS BEST GUESS.

JOE MADE HIS LIVING IN HOUSTON AS A TAXIDERMIST AND UNION IRONWORKER.

Joe and Helen settled in Houston. He joined the Ironworker's Local 84 apprenticeship program in June of 1947. Joe became a journeyman in August 1949, honorary member in October 1981, and lifetime retired member in January 1983.

The requirements for an ironworker were as rough and tumble as Patton's infantry, and Joe wouldn't have had any other type of job—fearlessness and courage on the inside and on the outside good physical conditioning, agility, and strength.

The apprentice tests were hard. There were three parts—physical, mental, and psychological. Failure on any part meant disqualification. The tests were given every three years, and if a man failed, he was out of luck. He had to wait for the next test.

There was also an age limit of 29. Anyone older than that had to find another line of work. Although there were no blacks in the union, it was not segregated. It was about 60 percent white, and the rest were American Indians.

Joe's knowledge of diverse, yet connected, subjects; his talents with his mind and hands and his many odd and interesting eccentricities made him well known in Houston.

Joe wrote a tribute, *"High Steel,"* to his co-workers on his last day on the job in 1980, and he would often recite his poetry. He would speak to college students in Houston on taxidermy, paleontology, geology, and his fossil collections because he was so widely read on many subjects. In addition to evolution and paleontology, he had a life-long passion for history and philosophy that tended to support his stoic agnosticism.

REQUIREMENTS FOR AN IRONWORKER

"**Good physical condition.** *The materials used for ironworking are heavy and bulky so above average physical strength is necessary. Agility and a good sense of balance are required. It is important to mention that an ironworker must be willing to work in high places, have a good sense of balance, and be alert to potential danger to themselves and others."*

After the war, Houston's economy boomed due to the expanding Texas oil industry, and Local 84 ironworkers worked on seemingly unlimited numbers of jobs on high office buildings, bridges, warehouses, and roads throughout the area. Joe preferred high steel. Local 84 was known for having the best apprentice facilities in the country and had over 1,100 apprentices attending classes by the 1970s. The apprentice facilities are still in use today with state-of-the-art updates to ensure that apprentices are the best in the field. When Ironworkers Local 84 celebrated its anniversary, the University of Houston history department identified the bold and daring in its research of Local 84 folk heroes, and Joe was one.

> **There are those who might someday say—**
> **'They don't deserve that big iron pay.'**
> **So come all you, who speak as such,**
> **Let's see if you dare to do as much.**
>
> —JOE HAAN, 1980

The Golden Gate Bridge, St. Louis Golden Arch, and Chicago's massive 110-story Sears Tower were all built by ironworkers.

Joe became proud of his craft as the most daring man to walk Houston's death-defying high steel tightrope. Nearly every structure built during Joe's post-war career—office towers, high-rise apartments, schools, sports stadiums, shopping malls, hospitals, bridges, industrial buildings—required the daring and rough-and-tumble skills of well-trained ironworkers, making them the most highly respected and best paid tradesmen in the construction industry.

Joe was proud he had helped build Houston's landmarks and shape the skylines of one of America's most rapidly growing cities. It was gratifying for him to be able to stand back, admire his work, and say, *"I helped build that!"* On many days—cold and warm, windy and calm—Joe worked high in the clouds erecting the skeletons of tall Houston skyscrapers. He set steel rebar in concrete to reinforce the framework and built complex steel ornamental structures, the taller and windier the better, as far as he was concerned.

Building the world's greatest steel structures became an amazing feat that fascinated Joe, especially the engineering. Most ironwork in Houston was done outdoors and could be carried on year-round except in very severe weather, but in many cases indoor work was coordinated with bad weather to keep people on the payroll. Safety devices such as nets, safety belts, and safety scaffolding were developed to reduce the risk of injury caused by the dangerous amount of climbing, balancing, and reaching overhead that was required.

Joe scoffed at weather delays and safety requirements even though he saw many steel workers fall to their deaths due to foolishness or a misstep. El Tigre Chiquita was known as the most fearless of them all, and he worked hard to live up to his nickname.

Joe set the standard for the daring Houston workers who walked the steel framework of tall buildings under construction—daredevils called structural ironworkers and known in the Texas press as *"cowboys of the skies."* Joe's usual job was to unload, erect, and connect fabricated iron structures and pieces to form the skeleton of a larger structure and to do this hundreds of feet off the ground in all types of weather.

Structural ironworkers would typically work on the construction of office towers and other tall industrial, commercial, and residential buildings, which became Joe's specialty. They would also work on bridges, stadiums, and prefabricated metal buildings from time to time. Joe always said he preferred *"High Steel"* and not the easy stuff like pre-cast beams, columns, and panels that could be easily assembled on the ground. Rigging was an integral part of the ironworking trade. Joe became an expert rigger, with a strong technical knowledge of fiber line, wire rope, hooks, skids, rollers, proper hand signals, and hoisting equipment. He tended to ignore training on government safety issues.

Joe and his fellow iron riggers would load, unload, move, and set machinery, structural steel, curtain walls, and other materials. They used power hoists, cranes, derricks, forklifts, and aerial lifts. Sometimes they lifted loads by hand with a series of block and tackle systems Joe first learned to use on the German farm. Welding and burning equipment were tools of the trade. Joe became an expert arc welder in the process, even artistic when he had the chance, which was frequent. Many of Joe's pieces of steel artwork survive, like the birds he artistically cut freehand from tempered steel, now in the Millersburg Schoolhouse Museum, with layers of carefully hammered feathers textured into the metal surface.

Over the years, *"high steel"* became part of Joe's life, granting him the same opportunities, problems, and issues he experienced during the war. Though offered promotions, Joe refused higher-paying supervisory positions where he could use his knowledge, but he refused to be the boss. Joe preferred to be a *"common soldier,"* like a *"Pfc grunt"* in the Army. And he was immediately ready to attack any type of prejudice or injustice. He was steadfastly intolerant of intolerance, especially when it came to fairness, equality, and fundamental human rights. But his hair-trigger alertness to danger made him a ticking timebomb.

Joe's poem "High Steel" appeared in The Ironworker magazine and is considered a classic in the ironworking trade, dedicated to his fellow devil-may-care ironworkers.

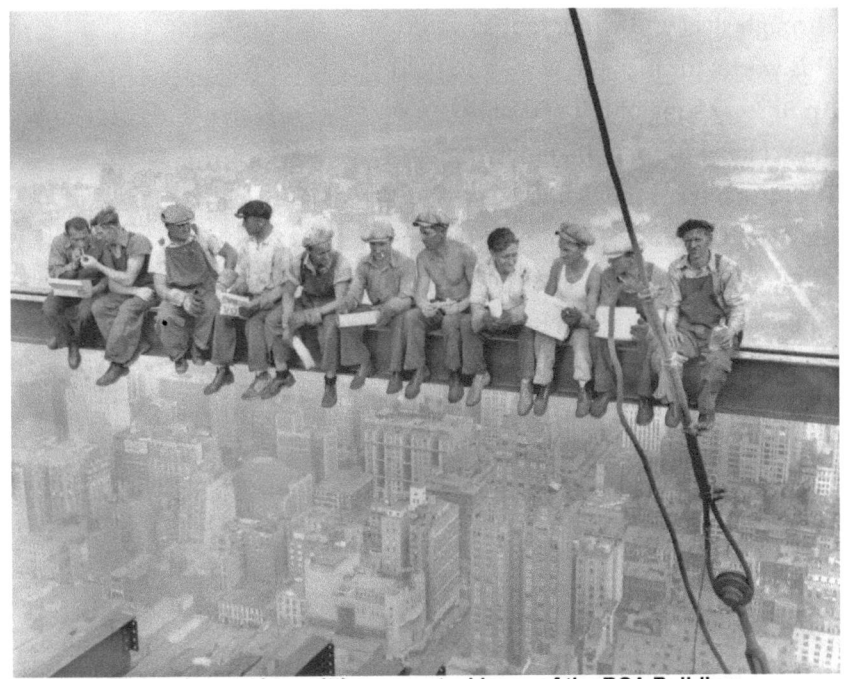

Eleven ironworkers sitting on a steel beam of the RCA Building, 850 feet above the ground during the construction of Rockefeller Center in Manhattan, New York City, September 20, 1932, photo public domain.

"HIGH STEEL" BY JOE HAAN 1980

In all the world of adventurous men,
The high steel boy is one of them.
On gird or truss or bridging high,
Many a hand has had to die.
Grab spinning hook, walk narrow beam,
This job's not what it might just seem.
Through sleet and wind, rain so cold,
This work's for men—few men so bold.
An unsung song of toil and pain,
In exchange for our small dollar gain.
Take a trip from the Golden Gate,
View high steel in the Empire State.
Wherever you may cast your eye,
You see their work up in the sky.
The many bridges that span the land,
Assembled by the ironworker's hand.

–Joe Haan

"Taking unnecessary risks is one of the first signs of war neurosis (PTSD)—nightmares, hallucinations come later."

DR. RIVERS, WW I

PTSD IN VETERANS

Globally, an estimated 354 million adult war survivors have PTSD and/or major depression. (*European Journal of Psychotraumatology,* 2019).

In one study of 1,938 veterans, a PTSD prevalence of about 14% was present in veterans who served in Iraq. (U.S. Department of Veterans Affairs).

A 10% prevalence of PTSD has been extrapolated for Gulf War veterans. (American Journal of Epidemiology, 2003).

About 30% of Vietnam veterans have had PTSD in their lifetime. (American Psychological Association, 1990).

DIAL 988 - TWENTY-FOUR HOUR SUICIDE PREVENTION HOTLINE

THEY CALLED HIM *"EL TIGRE CHIQUITO,"* THE LITTLE TIGER.

- **Joe worked as a taxidermist and union ironworker** for the rest of his working life.
- **His classic poem,** *"High Steel,"* was written for his co-workers on his last day on the job in 1980, and he would often recite his poetry.
- **Joe's knowledge of diverse yet connected subjects,** his many talents, and his interesting eccentricities made him well known in Houston.
- **He would show off his taxidermy** and fossil collections, discuss astronomy, paleontology, geology, evolution, religion, and his life-long passion for history.

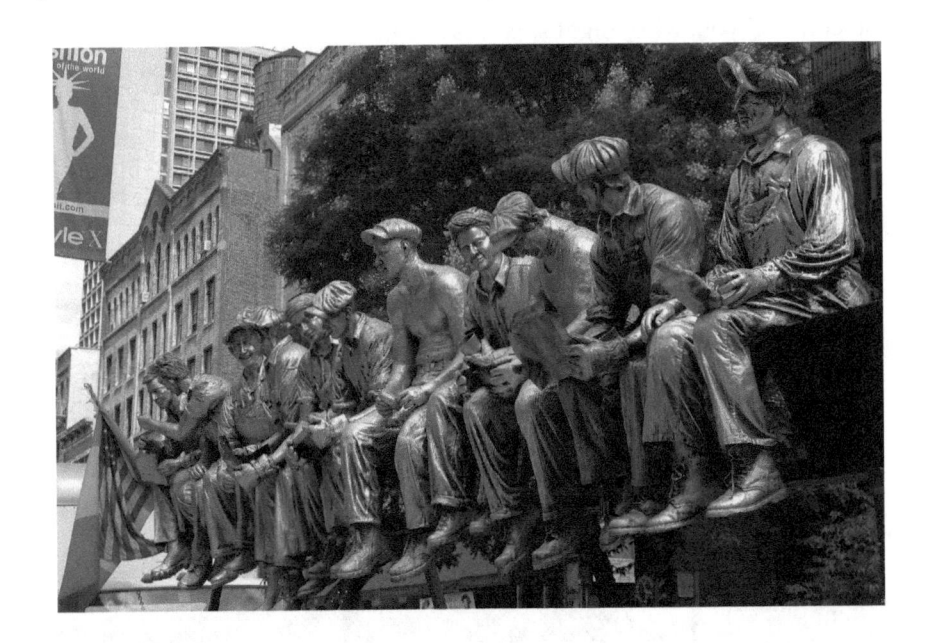

Veterans in Crisis

"HIGH STEEL" BY JOE HAAN 1980

And now, before all things are said,
Let us pay tribute to brothers dead.
For theirs was not to reason why,
They chose a task to death defy.
So they get the iron in their veins,
Risk life and limb for some few gains.
Up in the morn before break of day,
What fate decrees, no man can say.
Always walk iron with a little dread,
In exchange for this, our daily bread.
Where winds blow strong, men grow pale,
When caught up there in a raging gale.
There are those who might someday say—
"They don't deserve that big iron pay."
So come all you, who might speak as such,
Let's see if you dare to do as much.
Joe Haan

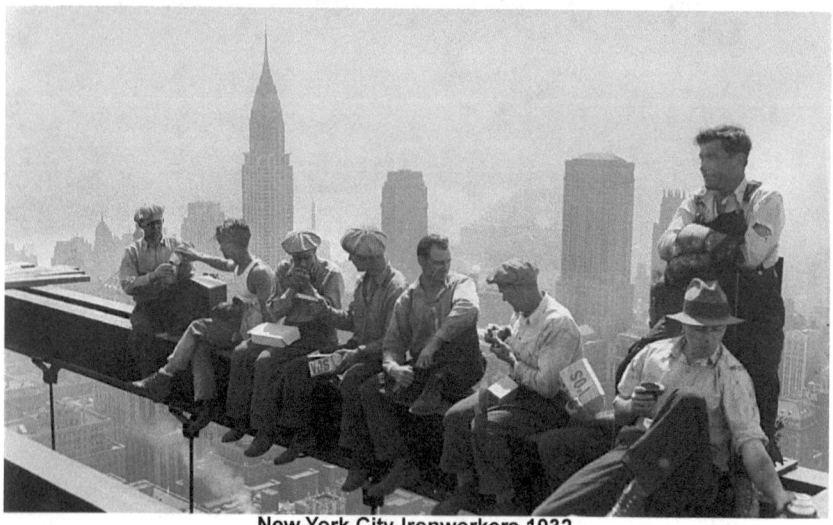

New York City Ironworkers 1932

UNION IRONWORKER

A job as an ironworker was about the only job Joe could have accepted and handled because of his fierce independence, drive, and constant demands. Joe was at his best when he worked alone on the hardest and most dangerous jobs.

The smart foremen soon got to know Joe and understand his ways because he was the best and fastest at what he did, and they knew it. But Joe worked strictly on his own terms. The number of times union foremen would tell him to slow down on the job, Joe couldn't say. He could tie steel several times faster than the average worker, and Joe would tell the other workers to get out of his way. That's how he always worked and why he was known as *"el Tigre Chiquito."*

There was never a better scout leader telling stories around the campfire.

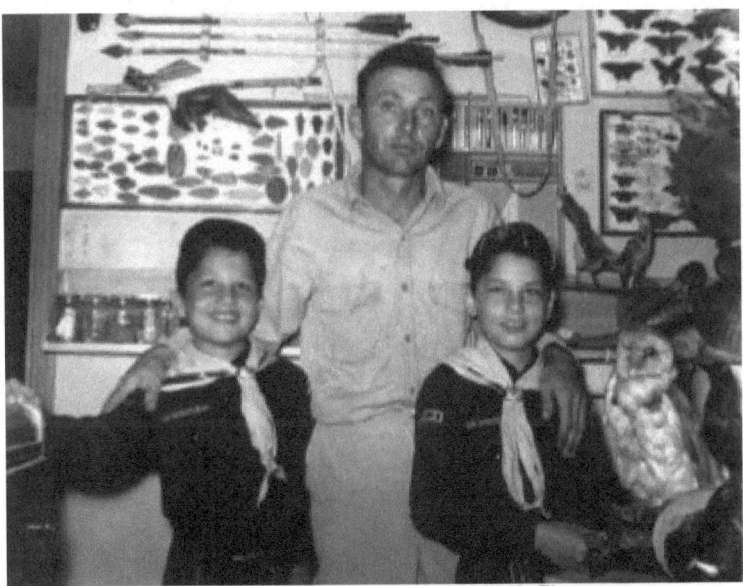

Sons Jack and James were born in 1948 and 1949. There was never a better scout leader telling stories around the campfire.

"The general theme of this work reflects chronic skepticism. Of that, I plead guilty. I owe one apology only, and that is to the devil, for lacking the ability to be more severe in my criticism of all organized religion."

– JOE HAAN

"THE WAR HAD A SERIOUS EFFECT ON JOE, OUR CRAZY UNCLE. AS KIDS WE WERE AFRAID OF HIM, BUT WE WERE ALSO FASCINATED."

A SUPERINTENDENT ON A CONSTRUCTION JOB PUT JOE TO WORK AS A LABORER. ONE OF THE FOREMEN HAD A GERMAN ACCENT. WHEN JOE WAS ON A SCAFFOLDING ABOUT 20 FEET UP IN THE AIR, THE FOREMAN YELLED SOMETHING AT JOE THAT MUST HAVE SOUNDED LIKE THE GERMAN FARMER. JOE JUMPED OFF THE SCAFFOLD AND LANDED ON TOP OF THE FOREMAN, RIPPING HIM TO PIECES. THEY THOUGHT JOE HAD KILLED THE GUY. JOE'S TEMPER SCARED THE HELL OUT OF EVERYONE ON THE JOB.

JOE WROTE IN HIS JOURNAL:

"AT TIMES I FIND MYSELF COMPLETELY ISOLATED IN MY THOUGHTS AND WITHOUT COMMUNICATION, AS IF I WERE AN ALIEN BEING, IN AN ALIEN WORLD, SOMEWHERE OUT IN INFINITY."

AFTER SUPPER JOE'S GUITAR AND HARMONICA

Joe would sing songs he wrote on the road and during the war, Woodie Guthrie style, sad and mournful, full of nostalgia and moral injury.

Joe had a huge trunk full of World War II memorabilia that he shipped from Germany and had sent to our house. It was a very large steamer trunk and had all sorts of German flags, bayonets, officer's swords, German helmet, Luger pistol, German medals, letters, money, coins, and other things he took off dead German soldiers. He had a German helmet with a bullet hole in it. The helmet was very well constructed with a full soft-cushioned leather liner in it with the name, "Schuck." He had a huge German battle flag in like-new condition. Joe told a story of how he and a buddy, blasting their way through a building in Germany, ended up with German jewelry and diamonds, But before they embarked for the States, they gave them up. The embarkation officer said, "All troops with looted goods go straight to prison."

I'm a young man that's gone away,
I've took a trip today.
To fight a war, and die, I may,
For what, I cannot say.
I know not what I'm fighting for,
It may be to open freedom's door,
So from our wounds our blood does pour,
While deafening cannons roar.

I loved the world, the world loves me,
Yes, just to live, to love and be.
Help me now, to strive and see,
Make all mankind free.

We are taught to take another life,

In painful, senseless insane strife,
We plead to you who sent us here,
Our crimes committed, you shall bear.

"Why Soldier, WHY" by Joe Haan, Germany, 1945.
(Capo 3 Fret Chord G+Ab)

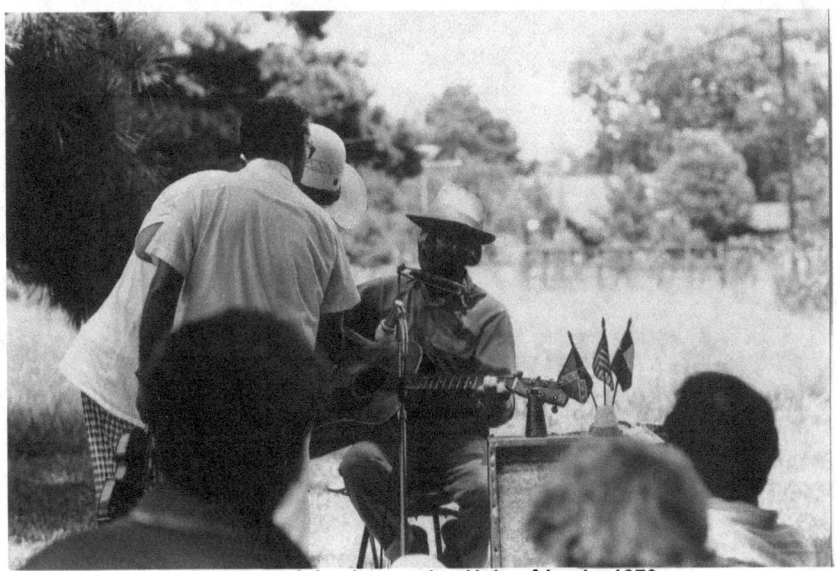

Joe entertaining Ironworker Union friends, 1970

Veterans in Crisis

TO BE EMPOWERED, THE DOC SAYS…

MANY PEOPLE WHO ARE HURTING CLING TO THE NOTION THAT THEY ARE UNWORTHY.

BECAUSE THEY SUFFER, THEY SOMETIMES ACT OUT OF THEIR SUFFERING.

THEY OFTEN DON'T BELIEVE THEY DESERVE LOVE AND HAPPINESS.

THEY THINK ONLY WHEN THEY HAVE "*GOTTEN MY ACT TOGETHER*" WILL THEY BE WORTHY OF KINDNESS.

OFTEN THE PERSON SAYING THIS MOST PERSISTENTLY IS OURSELF.

DON'T WAIT TO BE EMPOWERED.

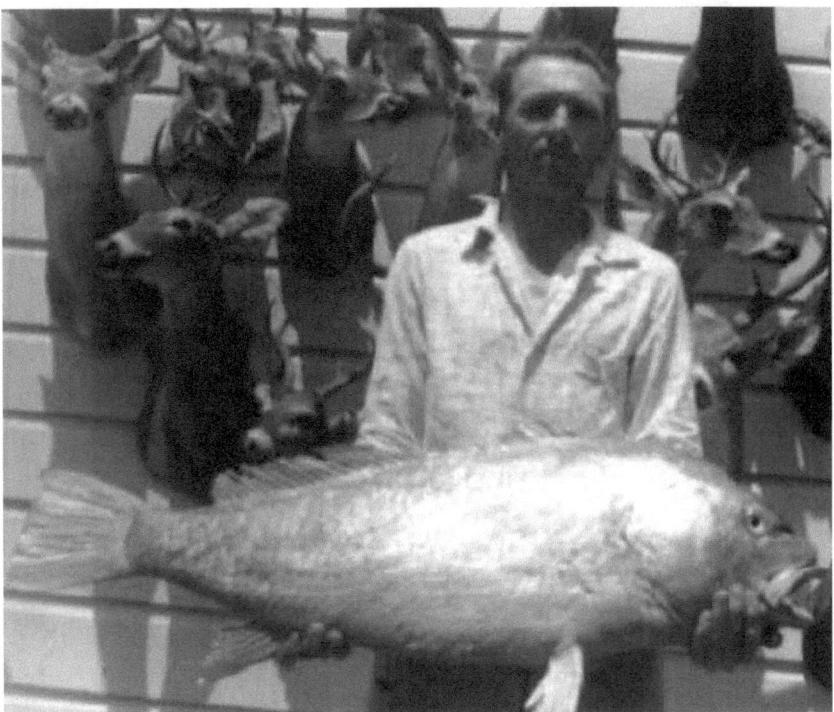

Joe with large black drum fish, 1959. Joe's motto was, "I bring 'em back to life."

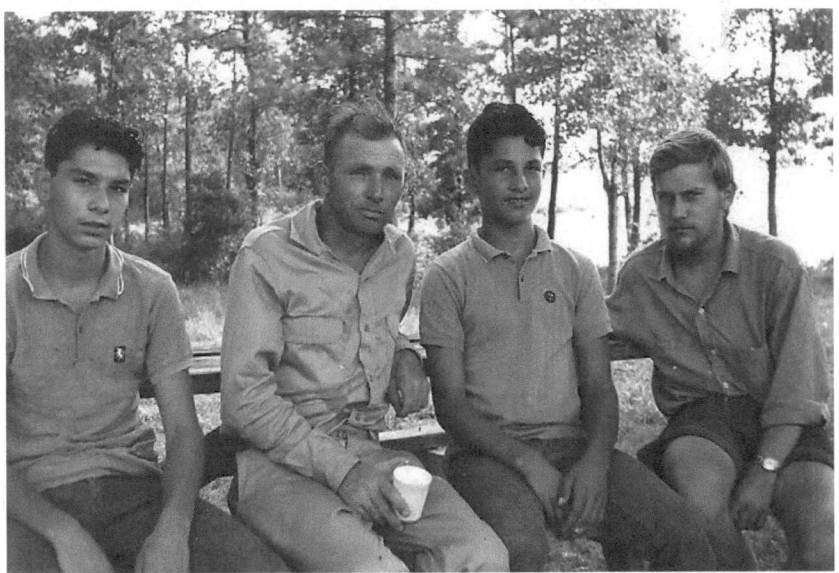

Son Jack, Joe, Son James, and friend Tim Carlson 1964

"I, and only I, take full responsibility for determining reality."

IRVIN D. YALOM

"Once the storm is over you won't remember how you made it through, how you managed to survive. You won't even be sure, in fact, whether the storm is really over. But one thing is certain. When you come out of the storm, you won't be the same person who walked in."

— HARUKI MURAKAMI
popular Japanese writer, collective trauma theme.

THE FOUR AGREEMENTS

1. *Be Impeccable With Your Word*
2. *Don't Take Anything Personally*
3. *Don't Make Assumptions*
4. *Always Do Your Best*

"Traumatized people feel chronically unsafe inside their bodies—the past is alive with a gnawing discomfort—they are constantly bombarded by visceral warning signs and signals."

"War is a Force that Gives us Meaning"

CHRIS HEDGES

> "We shall not cease from exploration
> And the end of all our exploring
> Will be to arrive where we started
> And know the place for the first time."
>
> **T.S. ELIOT**
> *"Little Gidding"*

EVENINGS WITH JOE

Joe loved talking philosophy, telling stories, and singing songs over a little Lone Star, Budweiser, and Sauterne. In addition to his scientific and artistic interests, Joe had a solid knowledge and understanding of the American Civil War based on in-depth reading and many trips to Civil War battlefields over the course of fifty years or more.

Through friends in Houston who shared his interests, Joe found the original unpublished Civil War letters of Corporal William Cunningham, a Wisconsin volunteer member of the Iron Brigade that was decimated on the morning of the first day at Gettysburg, July 1, 1863. Joe knew the story of the Iron Brigade, having first walked the battlefield of Gettysburg in the summer of 1938 on the very ground and woods where the Iron Brigade made its last stand against Lee's advancing Confederate Army.

William Cunningham's Civil War letters were written to his girlfriend Mary Parrish back home in Avoca, Wisconsin. They recount the pain, suffering, defeat, and tragedy he endured during the Civil War as a member of the 2nd Wisconsin Infantry, one of the few western regiments to serve *"back east"* with the Army of the Potomac.

The letters moved Joe because they told a universal story of a patriotic and idealistic young soldier caught up in events far beyond his control. He wrote to his girlfriend back home and expressed eternal hope and optimism, following defeat after successive defeat. Joe believed he had known William Cunningham as a fellow comrade-in-arms.

The William Cunningham letters reminded Joe of his wartime experience in France, Belgium, Luxembourg, and Germany, but Joe had survived his war, and William Cunningham had not. Joe seemed to understand what happened to William Cunningham and his best friend, Sergeant Spencer Train, that first day at Gettysburg in 1863.

Joe lived with a burden of guilt for having been spared in combat during the violence he experienced in 1944 and 1945. Joe had heard other World War II vets talk about a feeling of *"survivor guilt"* for having lived while their comrades had died.

Ambivalent feelings are expressed throughout Joe's poetry, especially in *"Ode to William Cunningham,"* where he describes William Cunningham in McPherson's Woods at the time of his final, fatal martial clash, as though Joe were present there beside the wounded corporal and best friend Sgt Spencer Train.

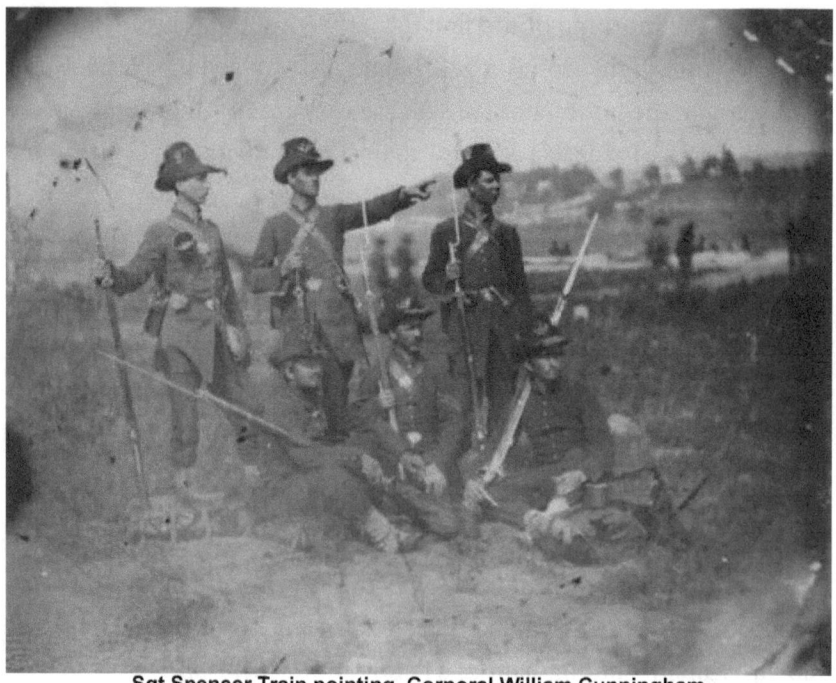

Sgt Spencer Train pointing. Corporal William Cunningham front row, center, kneeling.

ODE TO CORPORAL WILLIAM CUMMINGHAM

Artificer, 2nd Wisconsin Infantry, Iron Brigade, Army of the Potomac
1861-1863

By Joe Haan (Notebook II)

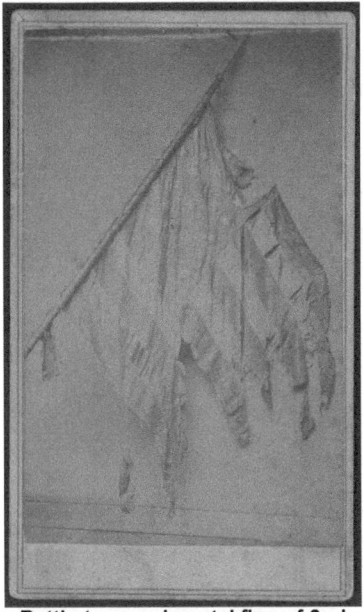

Battle-torn regimental flag of 2nd Wisconsin Infantry Regiment (Iron Brigade) damaged at the Battle of Gettysburg

He seemed to have an ancient sense of justice,
Reincarnated from some distant past,
A total abhorrence to subjugation, the binding of men,
In spite of the fact that he had made
But 20 short trips about the sun.
To all free-loving men, he knew,
No nation could exist, half slave, half free.

The sounds of far-off war trumpets
Amplified this message to William Cunningham,
So the angry guns would speak,
And many noble men
Would walk into the maw of death,
And endless bitter tears would flow
In half a million simple homes,
For so many young Wills would be no more,
Only known as the vast "Unknown,"
Lying in a desolate field, undignified in death.
Truly did they inherit the earth.

Private William Cunningham
Was unique in more ways than one:
In an age when the greater percentage
Of young men his age were ill-educated,
His power of expression stood out
With a rather limited vocabulary,
A certainty his intellectual achievement
Was recognized by his comrades in arms.

As war banners unfurled in the winds,
Martial tunes were struck in 1861,
Simple young farm boys
Congregated from near and far
Upon the parade ground
At Madison, Wisconsin.

And Oh, how their spines did tingle
In the limelight of history and public acclaim,
And would not history proclaim
They exemplified the very best in courage,
With a sense of justice that could not be equaled.
All willing martyrs, no conscripts these.

Red hot cannister and grape shot
Cut great swaths in their ranks
That first day at Gettysburg,
And after overwhelming pain, oblivion.
The Iron Brigade would be no more,
Only many vacant chairs,
And years of gnawing agony for loved ones.

Over this enigma of life
And sudden violent death,
For how does one reason out,
This wasting of human intellect,
The squandering of one
Who showed so much potential
For further achievement in any field?

Some men are priceless,
Others of little value whatsoever.
This contrast is self-evident on every hand;
Sometimes a gem occurs in a field of dirt—
For justice is an artificial thing,
Created by homosapien man
Out of the primordial past, from which he evolved,
Where no such thing as mercy or justice existed.

Even now, some men lay down their lives
On the altar of sacrifice,
For principles they feel
Are the only correct ones,
Though they may realize
They shall never pass this way again,
Manly unsung heroes, these,
No man yet, shall they displease,
With malice toward none, charity for all.

CIVIL WAR TRIPS WITH JOE

Over the years, Joe went on many Civil War trips to Pea Ridge and remote areas of Alabama, Mississippi, and Georgia. In 1974, just before going working in the Dominican Republic, Joe traveled to Washington, DC and tramped Civil War battlefields in Pennsylvania, Maryland, and Virginia.

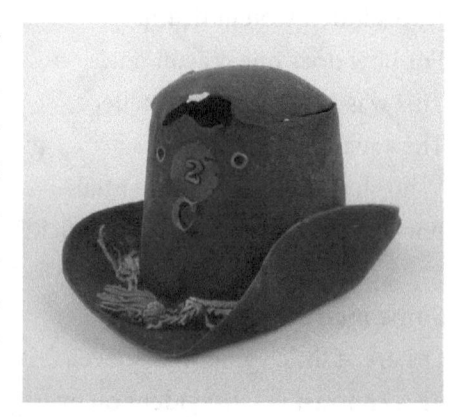

Joe was still very agile at the age of 56, and his audience at a Greek restaurant downtown Washington, DC couldn't believe his one-footed dance on stage with a belly dancer while biting his big toe on a dare.

Joe was always quick and agile like a cat and very strong—he said it was a family trait. He said that it had helped him survive over the years, along with his well-developed intuition. Joe said his intuition saved him several times during the war—subliminal warnings of impending danger he had learned to heed, causing him more than once to hit the deck just in time or refuse to volunteer for a dangerous patrol assignment. In the spring of 1997, the spirit of Joe led to a Civil War trip down the Mississippi River to Vicksburg. Joe loved the journey and the memories it evoked.

Remembering Joe at Vicksburg. Early in the month of April, they journeyed through the length and breadth of the State of Mississippi, first down the Great River to Hannibal, St. Louis, Fort Donnelson, then Shiloh and Memphis.

And further south in search of "Sam" Grant, along the Mighty Old Man River, banks overflowing with Minnesota waters, muddy, sprawling, meandering—a giant spill of melted snow, working its way to the Gulf of Mexico, and beyond, to evaporate and rise in wet and humid clouds with rain and snow, yet once again the process starts anew.

They saw the River, working and plodding its way past Vicksburg, Port Gibson, down the Natchez Trace, an ancient footpath linking Nashville to Natchez on the River. Moving ever southward over Emerald Mound, testament to early Mississippians who once resided and prospered along the fertile banks of the black-earthed Mississippi Delta, fertile northern soils washed by eons of erosion.

Moving again along the ancient Trace, through Jefferson to Natchez on the River, fragrant flowers, antebellum-style, colored azalea, dogwood, flowering April spruce, sleeping, resting with the dead.

Beginning slowly along the Trace, footsteps of a past long gone to Sam Grant's landing at Bruinsburg on the River, below Vicksburg's ramparts, running the gauntlet with 23,000 Yankee troopers, the largest amphibious operation in the history of the world before D-Day 1945.

Wending the way from Bruinsburg, back to Port Gibson, lunching at an unpainted country store, lazing in a napping noonday sun, they followed Sam Grant and 45,000 Midwest Yankees to the Battlefield of Raymond, northeastward, in the direction of Jackson, away from Vicksburg, Grant style, always victorious, through counties black and poor, black folk with unstained bloodlines, no mulattos these, turning west upon the foe, Confederate General Pemberton, wrapping him up at Champion Hill, the greatest battle of the American Civil War, some say.

Yet today—no marker, no memory, nothing to remind that something more than scrubby pine had ever ventured forth in an area known as Champion Hill, fifty-four thousand engaged in battle, the greatest perhaps, now overgrown and forgotten.

Then to the Big Black, a railroad trestle, a battle and a river crossing, the line of Confederate retreat into the City of Vicksburg, backed up against Old Man River, a siege—long, hot and dusty days—bombardments everlasting, scant food and rancid, rats as morsels cooked with pea ground bread, and final ignominious surrender to U. S. Grant on the Fourth of July, 1863, the same day as victory back east at Gettysburg.

Breaking the back of the Confederacy—forever—the Union saved, Old Man River free again to move its cargo up and down the Father of Waters, northern farmers, no longer hostage to move wheat to market, *"Free at last, free at last, thank God amighty we'se free, at last."*

And they moved ever northward, in further tribute to an Oxford Man of Letters. *"Faulkner drank,"* the neighbors said, *"His father too."* Moonshine bottles, 182 empties, in the Rowan Oak woodshed, Old Turkey and Jack Daniels when times were good, Moonshine good enough for sippin' on other, leaner days.

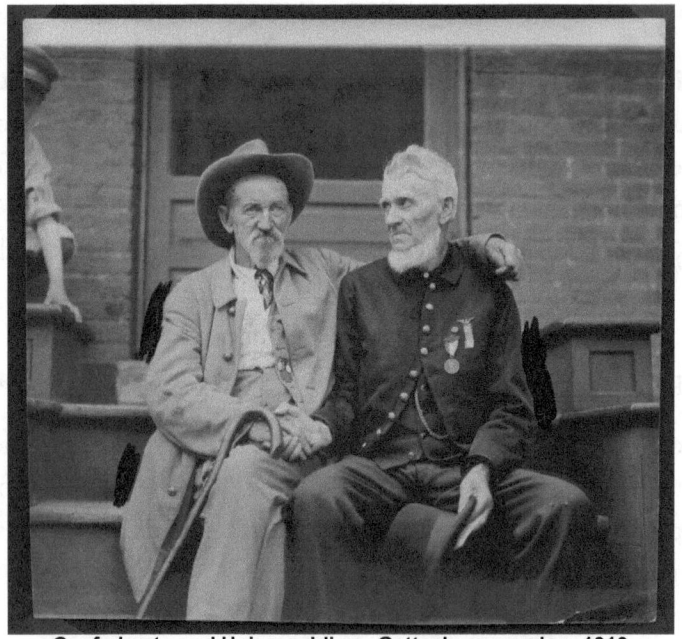

Confederate and Union soldiers, Gettysburg reunion, 1913

Approaching Rowan Oak, a pleasant country breakfast in the Coffeeville Café, a time warp—Billy Joel, the log cabin, a gentle April rain—a misty Saturday morning, bookstore on the Square, coffee, the Veranda, a football player, the Colts, Supreme Court Justice, Rebels, Ole Miss, faces, names, and Holly Springs.

A trip South, along the Mississippi, in the month of April, with Joe in spirit, seeing sights not seen by mortal eyes, except with Joe.

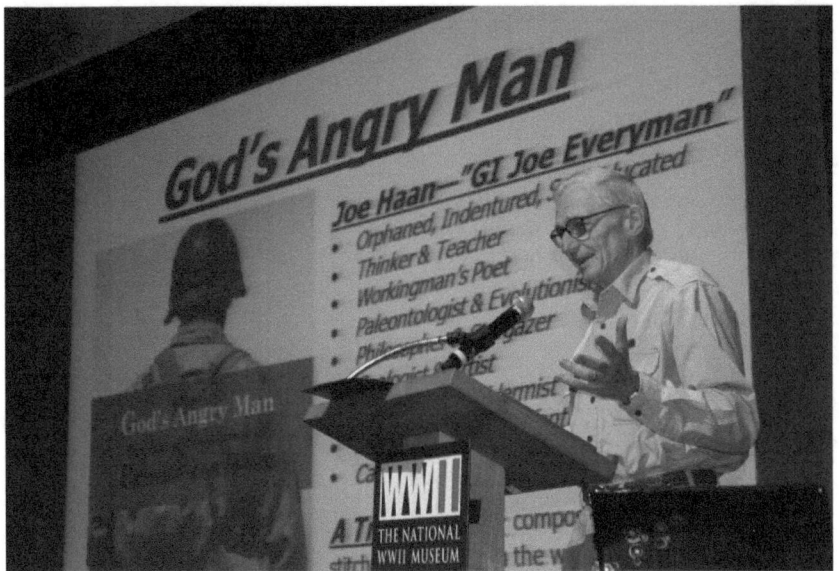

Colonel B. Wayne Quist, The National World War II Museum, 10-28-2010.

Veterans in Crisis

JOE LOVED LINCOLN

Lincoln's words echo with meaning yet today for every veteran and every American.

> *"...to care for him who shall have borne the battle and for his widow and his orphan."*

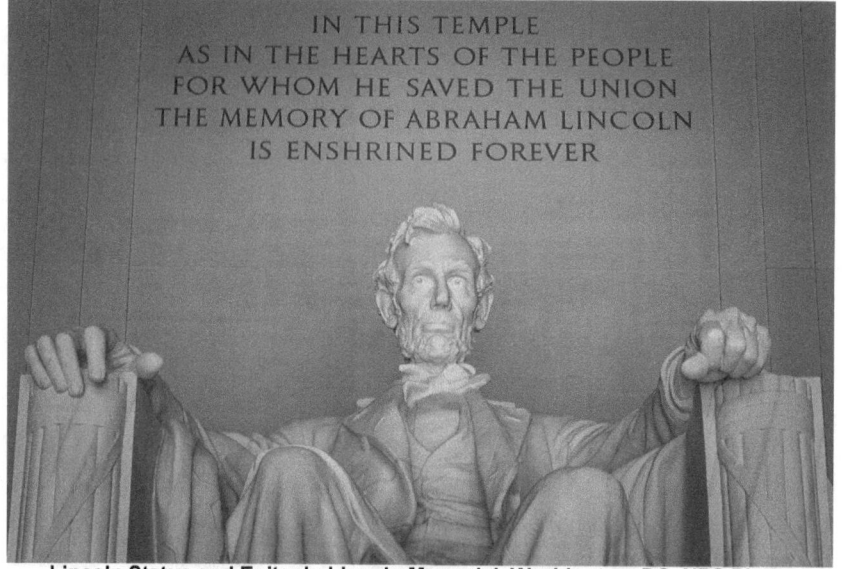

Lincoln Statue and Epitaph. Lincoln Memorial, Washington, DC. NPS Photo

"In this temple as in the hearts of the people for whom he saved the Union, the memory of Abraham Lincoln is enshrined forever."

LINCOLN'S SECOND INAUGURAL ADDRESS

March 4, 1865

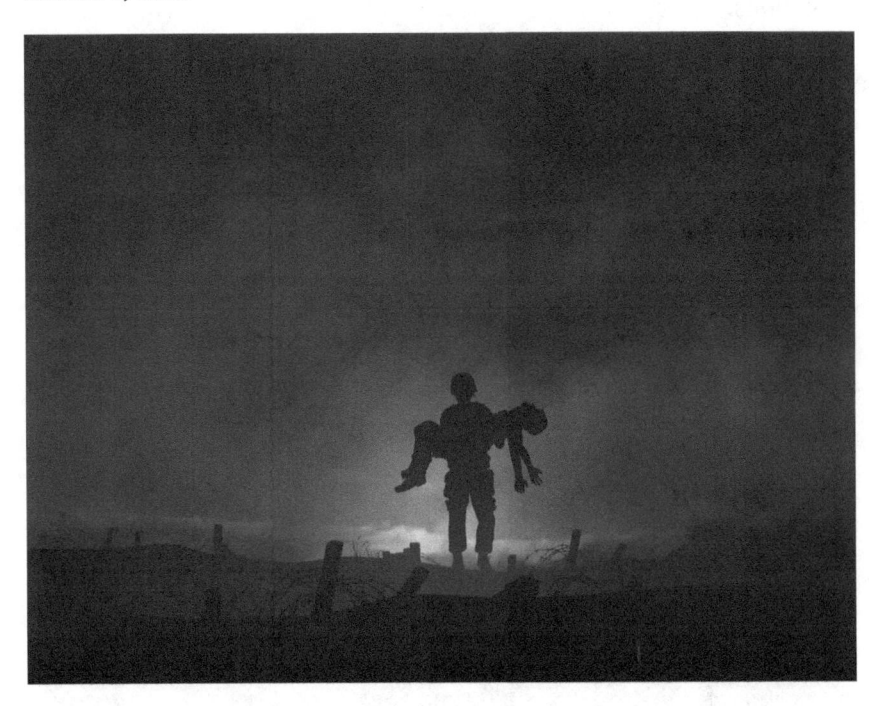

Fondly do we hope, fervently do we pray, that this mighty scourge of war may speedily pass away.

Yet, if God wills that it continue until all the wealth piled by the bondsman's two hundred and fifty years of unrequited toil shall be sunk and until every drop of blood drawn with the lash shall be paid by another drawn with the sword as was said three thousand years ago so still it must be said 'the judgments of the Lord are true and righteous altogether.

With malice toward none with charity for all with firmness in the right as God gives us to see the right let us strive on to finish the work we are in to bind up the nation's wounds, to care for him who shall have borne the battle and for his widow and his orphan, to do all which may achieve and cherish a just and lasting peace among ourselves and with all nations.

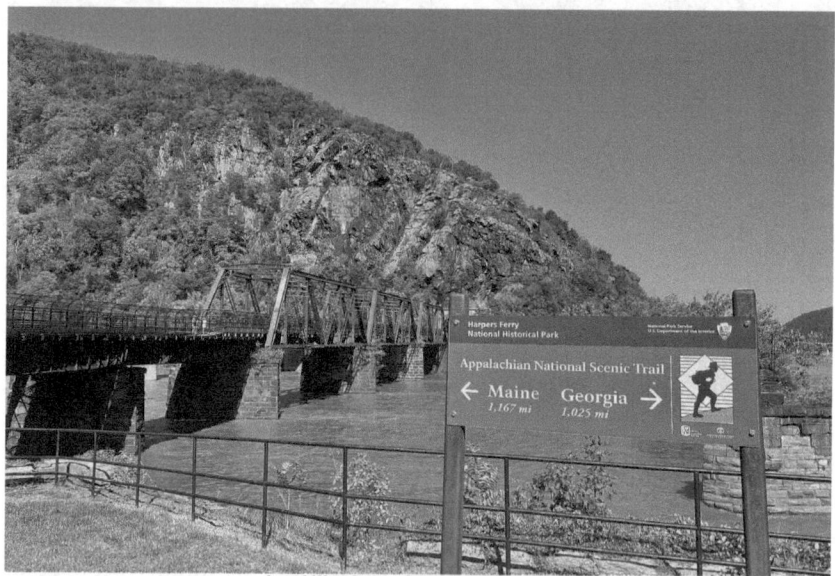

Joe Hiked the Appalachian Trail

A SYMPOSIUM WITH JOE

Journalist Tom Brokaw wrote about the bravery and distinctiveness of the World War II veterans in his book *"The Greatest Generation."* Joe and his comrades fought and died to save the world from the 20th century's deadly totalitarian movements.

Now another life cycle following the Greatest Generation is mopping up the immoderation of the *"Me Too"* generation, seeking to bring the world back into equilibrium as Joe and his generation did in their time. As *"god's angry man,"* Joe would have written of the excesses of the 21st century in words he would have shouted loudly to the world as the last iconoclast.

An evening with Joe was always memorable. Joe couldn't talk to you without touching you, manhandling you, his hand on your shoulder, on your head, or holding both your arms. There was no escape. He had your total attention and he dominated. Joe always spoke loudly because his hearing had been impaired by World War II artillery. As he grasped your arms, you could feel his intensity, see his furrowed brow, deep-sun-burned creases along his cheeks, and riveting blue eyes. Joe was mesmerizing. Everything about Joe commanded your total attention, and he got it. The dialogue and conversations developed a rhythm of their own and the subjects would run the gamut from survival to metaphysical.

An evening with Joe might start with a depiction or reenactment of one of the great battles of history—Alexander the Great in Persia, Julius Caesar in Gaul, or General Patton and Joe at the Battle of the Bulge along the Sûre River a few miles south of Bastogne.

He might follow with a lengthy dissertation on Joe's version of the Origin of the Species: *"In the beginning, Man created god ... you'll never look at an ape in the same way again."*

Before long, the guitar and harmonica would come out. Joe would sing his songs, and always *"This Land Is Your Land"*—he loved Woody Guthrie. Then a Jack London story, building a fire in the Arctic winter of young minds, which might lead to Robert Service and *"The Cremation of Sam McGee."* He would follow with a lecture on igneous, sedimentary and metamorphic rocks, never-ending questions and his answers:

"Want to know how to skin a lynx without cutting its eyelids?" He told us. *"Want to hone the sharpest knife in the world?"* He showed us. *"Want to know the best way to hop a moving freight train? Well, let me tell you,"* and he would, as more answers to his questions continued: *"This is how you make a Clovis spearpoint like Helen's forefathers did 12,000 years ago. You have to watch the size of your flakes as you chip away the flint. And this is how to stay alive in a freezing foxhole with your dead enemy as your only companion."*

Then, as we would step outside; the inevitable toast would ring loudly into the hot and sweaty Houston night: *"Hold your glasses steady boys, for this life, it's a pack of lies—Drink to the dead already, boys, and Hurrah for the next man who dies!"*

Now, here's the wrestling part. At some point in the evening, you were sure to find yourself by Joe's lush garden in the back yard. Suddenly you're flat on your back in an instant, looking up at the stars. It's Joe, practicing his karate hold on you. Just as suddenly, he throws the Korean Deathlock on you, and there's absolutely no escape until you cry, *"Uncle."*

The curriculum at Joe's symposium was both mental and physical, and as the night wore on, the Sauterne and Lone Star lubricated the sense that we were at the center of the universe participating in an ancient ritual, a symposium with the grand master, an unforgettable human being, a remarkable teacher. We were his fortunate students.

As you entered the front room of Joe's house, you were immediately greeted by a six-foot high Tyrannosaurus Rex dinosaur Joe had molded from clay. Throughout the house, the walls were covered with more than a hundred stuffed animals and fish, every kind of deer, javelinas, many varieties of snakes, shark jaws, antelope, hawks, eagles, and rats.

Joe had turned his house into a natural history museum with stuffed animals and reptiles of all sizes and shapes; beautiful butterflies and poisonous insects; lifetime collections of minerals varying from meteorites to semi-precious stones found or mined by Joe over the years; Civil War Minié balls, hundreds of arrowheads, strange metals, and flags; coin, stamp, and currency collections; German bayonets, helmets, flags, and Lugers he brought home as war souvenirs. If Joe identified with it, the rare item was in one of his many collections throughout the house.

Driving by Joe's house in North Houston, no one would ever suspect that its occupant was so much different from the neighbors. Joe bought the one-story rambler in the 1950s for $7,500 and it was still worth about that when it was demolished to make room for a freeway around the turn of the century.

By the 1970s, the white middle class neighborhood had evolved into an all-black, desperately poor enclave with an economy based on drugs. Every night, a procession of vehicles would line up on Landor Lane, stopping two houses down from Joe. An 8-10 year-old kid would run out to the car and collect the money. The car would pull forward to the house next door to Joe's, and another young kid would run out to deliver the drugs to the waiting car, which immediately sped away. It was a business, a well-greased system, and it went on all night, every night.

After a break-in when someone stole his guns, Joe installed steel bars on every window and heavy steel doors and locks. The neighborhood left the strange old taxidermist/ironworker alone. Joe was friendly with his black neighbors, but he was white. They wondered to themselves why any sane white man would choose to live in a place where all the neighbors dreamed of escaping, but couldn't, as they were trapped in poverty.

But behind those barred windows was a man who empathized with their plight more than they would ever know. He was a man trying to make sense of a chaotic universe, a man who wrestled daily with man's inhumanity to his fellow man. Joe knew we are all children of our history, and he knew he belonged there at his first home on black Landor Lane. He chose not to leave because it was home, and he felt his neighbors' poverty and felt their crying needs, which he tended to.

The latest of many drug murders in Joe's neighborhood had occurred the night before we arrived in Houston on one of our many visits. The ambulance had come and awakened Joe late at night. The next morning, Joe walked across the street to the park where the murder had taken place. There on the grass was a mass of blood and a clump of human brains, the dead man's brains that had been literally blown out of his head, but too messy for the busy ambulance crew to pick up and remove with the dead body.

Joe went home and came back with a shovel and bucket. With care, he put the man's brains in the bucket and carried them to a quiet corner of the park. He buried them in an unmarked grave, pondering all the while the senseless loss of human life. Joe had been there before, on grave duty in France, after the Battle of the Bulge, later in Germany. Another senseless death, another night in the Houston ghetto.

By the 1970s, North Houston resembled the third world, as we would witness when Joe showed us around his neighborhood. He took us into an all-black convenience store with very few goods for sale—just pop, candy, cigarettes, and a large screened-in beer and liquor area.

The clerk was stationed like a sentry at the front door, sitting on a stool. Directly behind her was a large, tattooed man who didn't smile, with a sawed off shotgun chained to his left arm.

Then we walked across the street to Joe's all-black local bar. Joe went there frequently enough that the patrons all knew him by name. They knew that he was a little different but not much else. Few white men would dare venture into this all-black bar. Except for occasional guests Joe would show around, no other white person ever dared enter the neighborhood, much less the local bar. But it was OK that we were there with Joe; that was the subliminal message in one of the most interesting bars ever.

You had to know it was a bar. There were no signs anywhere advertising its name or type of business. The walls were made of recycled plywood. The ceiling was a blue tarp that served as the roof. The bar itself was made of three 55-gallon steel barrels with two-by-twelve planks serving as the bar top. Patrons sat on metal folding chairs around cheap card tables. The entire nature of the bar gave the impression that it could pack up and move out in a few minutes.

The floor never had to be swept because it was dirt. Lou Rawls albums played on the 78 RPM record player, *"Breaking My Back Instead of Using My Mind"* and *"I'd Rather Drink Muddy Water."* We ordered three Lone Stars from the obliging bartender who walked over to a ten-year-old kid behind the bar and handed him some money. The kid returned a few minutes later with three beers he purchased at the convenience store with the shotgun guard we had just left across the street.

This was Joe's world, his own sociology laboratory. He openly shared it with us, in sorrow at the human condition but also proud that he was able to live and survive there. It was home, his first and last home.

Joe had worked with steel all his working life. Through an ironworker companion, he came by some exceptionally high quality steel with just the properties he needed to make the sharpest blade in the world. He took it from there, heating the steel to cherry red and carefully cooling it in gentle oil baths. Then he would pound it time and again to perfectly align the atoms. Through time, trial, and self-taught metallurgy, Joe developed what he called *"the sharpest knife in the world."* His favorite demonstration was to take a silk scarf and throw it in the air. As it passed gently over the stationary knife, drifting silently, the scarf was cut in half.

We pondered the sharpest knife in the world late one evening when the knife was at my throat. Joe was wound up about some injustice that needed correcting when he grabbed the knife, put it up to my throat, and said the bastards should be decapitated. At the time, I didn't realize this was simply Joe's way of making his point. Putting down the knife, he kissed me on the cheek. He reassured me that he meant no harm to his nephew, but all evildoers should beware. We've often thought of the sharpest knife in the world over the years.

Often, lying in bed at night before sleep falls, I recall the first time Joe took us on a trip through the universe. It was a dark summer night, and we were lying on the grass in Joe's backyard when the stars were amazingly bright. Joe knew all the names of the ancient constellations. To him, they were like old friends. He knew their locations by time of day and month of year. He would say:

"Take a trip with me through the universe." The light we see from the stars is ancient light. You have to understand the speed of light to give the universe any meaningful perspective. The speed of light is 186,000 miles per second, so it takes but one and one half seconds for light from the moon to reach Earth; two minutes from Venus to Earth, four minutes from Mars, Jupiter thirty minutes, and Saturn one hour. Neptune is four hours away. The Oort cloud with a trillion comets is one light year

away or about 5.9 trillion miles, while our sun is just eight minutes away.

"Our nearest neighbor star is Alpha Centauri"—you see it there on the southern horizon; it's just four light years distant. Man will go there some day. The Pleiades, the ancient Greeks' Seven Sisters, is 375 light years away. Remember, you're traveling at 186,000 miles per second. The Andromeda galaxy is two million light years distant. Get it?

"You're traveling at 186,000 miles per second for two million years" to get to Andromeda. The light we see from it tonight left there when man first started to walk upright. Further out, light coming from the Hercules cluster of galaxies 500 million light years away left millions of years before dinosaurs walked the Earth. The end of the known universe is out there some ten billion light years plus. The light that left there with the Big Bang is over five billion years older than our solar system.

"With trillions of stars in the universe" how many planets are there and how many of those planets have life? It would be the height of conceit to believe there's only one here on Earth. And what universes might lie beyond? Could we even calculate or fathom their distance with the speed of light as our crude and puny yardstick? Our Earth is in an outer spiral arm of our galaxy, the Milky Way, which has as many as a billion stars in it. Our known universe probably has as many as a billion galaxies. And remember, our galaxy, the Milky Way, is 100,000 light years across.

"Astronomers believe that at the center of each galaxy is a black hole" created by the death of a giant star. The black hole feeds and grows by consuming all that falls within its sphere of influence, its gravitational field. It will be our ultimate end, our oblivion, to fall prey to our own black hole, some billions of man-years hence. We, all of this, everything you see, will be drawn irretrievably closer and closer to the black hole in our galaxy. That is our destiny.

"At the point we pass the event horizon"—the moment the gravitational pull of our black hole takes over, the point of no return—at that instant, you and I and all we know, all of this around us, will be swallowed by the black hole. Within seconds, we will arrive at oblivion, the Great Singularity. Nothing passes the Great Singularity except pieces of atoms and fragments of light. It's all gone, everything! There is no way out."

Joe would say, *"The time will come when, discovery after discovery, science will reveal the secrets of the universe and man's place in it."*

Was the black hole at the center of our galaxy a metaphor for life as Joe had come to know it? If we are the totality of our genetic blueprint and our life experiences, then the essence of Joe is the spirit that drives us on, to wonder at it all.

We owe much to our Uncle Joe, as many of his genes predispose our curiosity, skepticism, sense of adventure, humanity, and mostly, our wonder of it all.

Joe, we'll meet you at the Great Singularity. – Joe's nephews Paul and Wayne Quist.

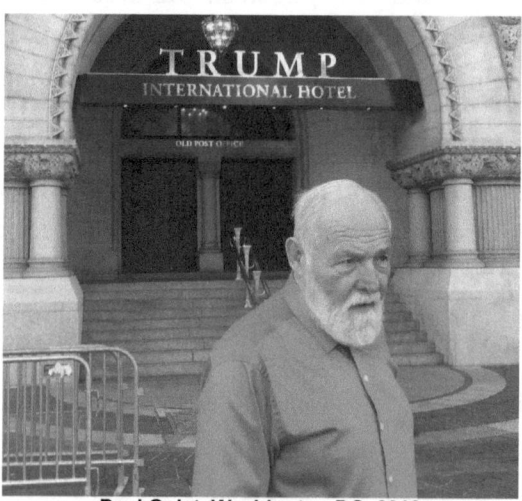

Paul Quist, Washington DC, 2019

"The unleashed power of the atom has changed everything save our modes of thinking and we thus drift toward unparalleled catastrophe."

ALBERT EINSTEIN

Veterans in Crisis

TO BE EMPOWERED, THE DOC SAYS...

"THE MILITARY ETHIC ACCEPTS THE NATION STATE AS THE HIGHEST FORM OF POLITICAL ORGANIZATION AND RECOGNIZES THE CONTINUING LIKELIHOOD OF WAR AMONG NATION STATES ... IT EXALTS OBEDIENCE AS THE HIGHEST VIRTUE OF MILITARY MEN ... IT IS, IN BRIEF, REALISTIC AND CONSERVATIVE." **SAMUEL HUNTINGTON, "THE SOLDIER AND THE STATE, NY: VINTAGE 1964, PAGE 79.**

"A WAR TO PROTECT OTHER HUMAN BEINGS AGAINST TYRANNICAL INJUSTICE; A WAR TO GIVE VICTORY TO THEIR OWN IDEAS OF RIGHT AND GOOD, AND WHICH IS THEIR OWN WAR, CARRIED ON FOR AN HONEST PURPOSE BY THEIR FREE CHOICE,—IS OFTEN THE MEANS OF THEIR REGENERATION."

"A MAN WHO HAS NOTHING WHICH HE IS WILLING TO FIGHT FOR, NOTHING WHICH HE CARES MORE ABOUT THAN HE DOES ABOUT HIS PERSONAL SAFETY, IS A MISERABLE CREATURE WHO HAS NO CHANCE OF BEING FREE, UNLESS MADE AND KEPT SO BY THE EXERTIONS OF BETTER MEN THAN HIMSELF."

THE SPOILER MAN

Upon a planet, in time there grew,
A parasite-like, most hungry shrew.
It had two arms, a leg, a head,
Mother Earth will take them dead.
They covered her from head to girth,
With concrete substance, little worth.
Drove huge drills right through her skin,
To see just what might lie within.
There they found the gold called oil,
To cover fertile land and soil.
Spoil and ruin, all that would grow,
No more grain, to reap and sow.
Burned her hide with many fires,
Defiled her streams, pollution sired.
Changed the atomic nature of things,
So total destruction—that, it brings.
Mountains high of plastic dung,
On once verdant land, is flung.
Good ground covered with fancy stone,
To mark the place of dirty bone.
Once the air, so fine and sweet,
Corrupts now, what we daily eat.
Oh, Mother Earth, you must revolt,
Condemn this spoiler as we molt.
Keep that black and slimy ooze
Within the ground, or we shall lose.
Eradicate from your broad land,
This destructive holy band.

–Joe Haan (Book II, #24)

Veterans in Crisis

A WORD OF CAUTION FROM JOE, 1990

Pondering the future . . .

> *"As man marches down the endless corridor of time, to an unpredictable future, he shall either walk in the sun or return to the primitive darkness that was his past."*

> *"In the vastness of the sea of space, time is lost in an endless race."*

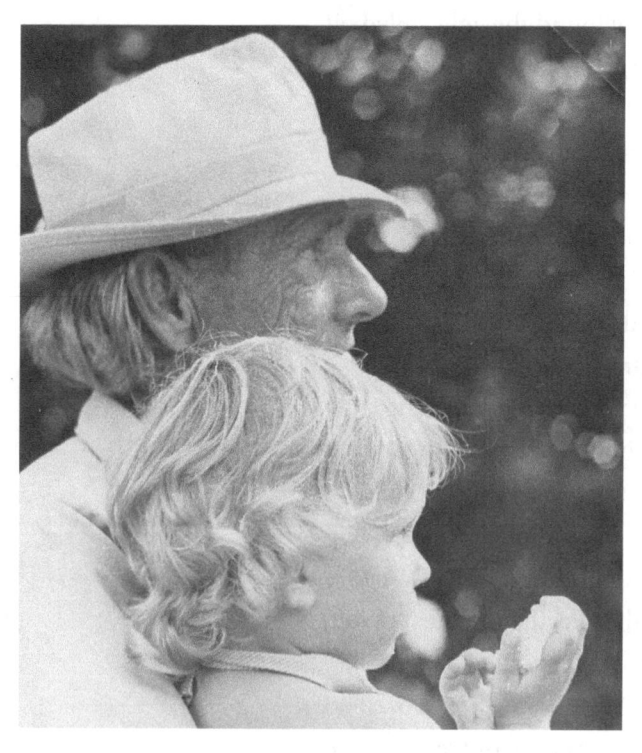

– JOE HAAN

JOE'S EPILOGUE

Joe died at the VA Hospital in Houston on January 7, 1992 from heart failure. He would have turned 74 in February. He had a 100% disability rating from the Veterans Administration, almost totally deaf from an ear drum broken by artillery. Helen sold the house on Landor Lane and eventually returned to her native Oklahoma to live with relatives. Joe's oldest son, Jack, lives in San Antonio where he has worked as a master carpenter. He has one daughter, Nave, Joe's only grandchild. Joe's youngest son, James, lives near Sacramento where he has worked as a building contractor, champion fish carver, and spiritual fishing guide in the remote Sierras. James and Jack both served in the Air Force.

Joe's epilogue is a short statement that summarizes the fate of the characters in this drama of life—namely Joe—and this brings us back to memories of the many times Joe toasted "the Bird" as he recited the old poem he loved, *"Mr. Flood's Party."* Joe met many Eben Flood characters on the road when he was riding the rails in the 1930s and later in Houston's Skid Row District. Many of them, like Joe, never had a birthday party or attended a party of any type in their lives.

Every Christmas in his later years, Joe would go downtown Houston where vagrants congregated to stay warm, and he became known as *"The Iron Man"* who handed out money to the homeless. *"Throw a nickel on the drum, save another drunken bum,"* was Joe's slogan. When asked by a Houston news reporter why he also gave free wine to winos at Christmas, Joe's honest response was, *"Because that's what they want."*

Joe often saw many Eben Floods on Houston's Skid Row, and he kept going back, especially in his retirement years. Joe ran across Edwin Arlington Robinson's poetry in one of America's libraries when he was on the road in the 1930s—homeless, alone, always broke—and every time he had a chance to take a drink of something potent, he would inevitably toast old Mr. Eben Flood and *"the Bird."* In his bones, Joe felt he knew Eben as a kindred soul, a brother.

Joe knew Mr. Flood from the feeling he got from Robinson's austere style and bleak subject matter. Mr. Flood appealed to Joe's sensitivity to human pain and suffering because he had endured so much of it—psychological, emotional, and physical pain, as well as anguish and suffering.

Visiting old slave quarters in Savannah or Charleston during his Civil War expeditions reminded Joe of his time at the Owatonna Orphanage and on Cobb Creek back in Minnesota amid the loneliness of the German farm. He shared their slave experience. He knew how they felt, beaten and worn from the ravages of pain, not being free. Joe would recite:

>"*Thank god for the solitude and beauty of nature,*
>*Thank god for the bountiful stars in the skies,*
>*Thank god for people like Mr. Eben Flood—*
>*May he rest in peace—and may he party on,*
>*In his 'valiant armor of scarred hopes outworn.'*
>*"Like Roland's ghost winding a silent horn …*
>*He raised again the jug, regretfully,*
>*And shook his head, and was again alone.*
>*There was not much that was ahead of him,*
>*And there was nothing in the town below—*
>*Where strangers shut the many doors*
>*That many friends had opened long ago."*
>
>*Joe's beloved poem, "Mr. flood's Party" by Edwin Arlington Robinson 1869-1935*

Dylan Thomas, Welch poet, 1914 – 1953
And death shall have no dominion.

>*Dead men naked they shall be one*
>*With the man in the wind and the west moon;*
>*When their bones are picked clean and the clean bones gone,*
>*They shall have stars at elbow and foot;*
>*Though they go mad they shall be sane,*
>*Though they sink through the sea they shall rise again;*
>*Though lovers be lost love shall not;*
>*And death shall have no dominion.*

Paul's epistle to the Romans (6:9), The Poems of Dylan Thomas. Reprinted by permission New Directions Publishing Corporation.

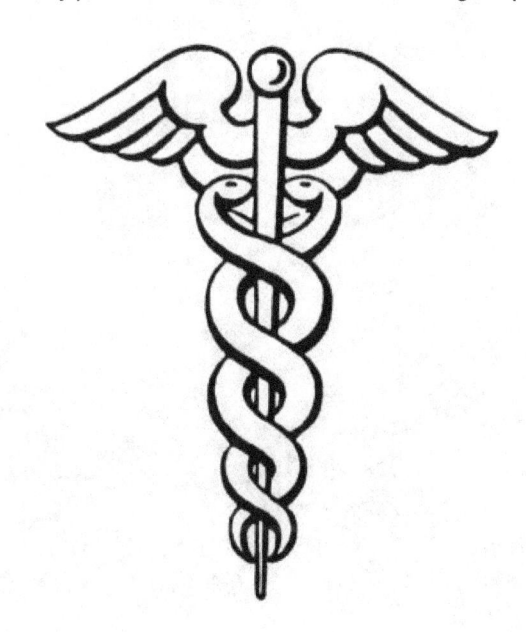

TIPS TO HELP WITH AN ANXIETY ATTACK

Look around you – use your senses: 5-4-3-2-1

> 5. Find five things you can see
> 4. Find four things you can feel
> 3. Find three things you can hear
> 2. Find two things you can smell
> 1. Find one thing you can taste

This is called "*grounding*." It can help when you feel you may have lost all control of your surroundings.

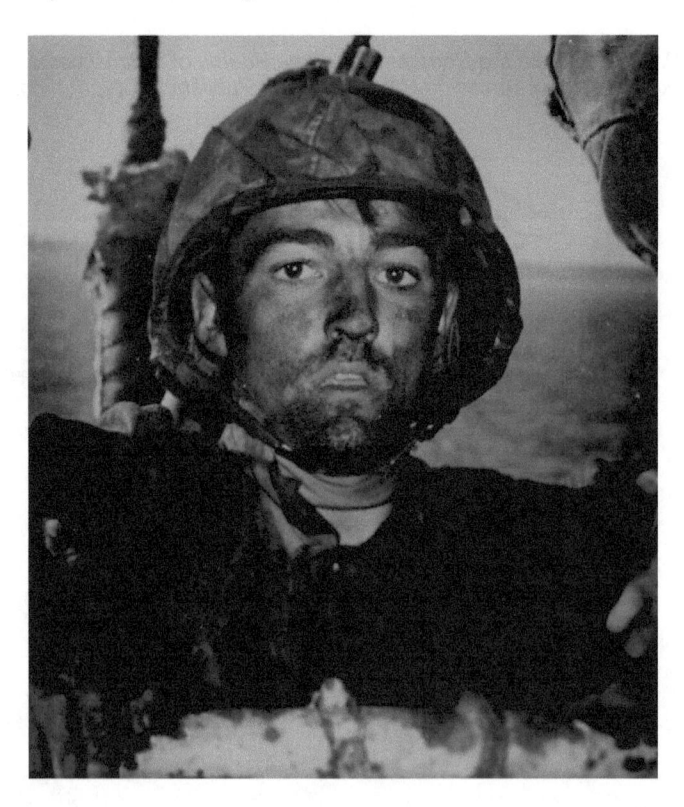

JOE'S WORDS OF WISDOM

"As man marches down the endless corridor of time, to an unpredictable future, he shall either walk in the sun or return to the primitive darkness that was his past." —Joe Haan, Houston, Texas, 1980

"What the world needs is more men that can be kind, to cultivate more true creativeness, and far less destruction." —Joe Haan, Alsace-Lorraine, France, 1944

"Far more galaxies there be, than fishes in the deep, dark sea. In the vastness of the sea of space, time is lost in an endless race." —Joe Haan, Houston, Texas, 1980

"It is clear to me the majority is always wrong." —*Joe Haan, Houston, Texas, 1980*

"Suffering makes men think; thinking makes men wise." —Joe Haan, Houston, Texas, 1980

"The lessons of life on Earth are these—to live, mankind must adapt; the species must evolve, to thus survive; for written in the code of mankind's DNA, immutable imprints of survival there reside. —Joe Haan to Paul Quist, 1974

"I was spawned of the Tree of Life and ate the fruit with little strife ..." —Joe Haan, Houston, Texas, 1980

"When all your atoms have finally fled, then you have found an eternal bed." —*Joe Haan, Houston, Texas, 1974*

"Trouble not the mind with fearsome fantasy, create not more dissembling mystery, so reason may drive all fear away, and destroy man's ignorance in this, our day." —Joe Haan, Houston, Texas, 1980

"Sometimes man is so completely confounded by the enigma of life that

he attempts to escape into a cocoon of myth and falsity, never to emerge into the light of knowledge." —Joe Haan, Alsace-Lorraine, France, 1944

"Man made thunder in my ears, tale of death is what one hears. Lightning flash within my eye, giant guns light up the sky." —Joe Haan, Alsace-Lorraine, France, 1944

"Under the roots of trees, dead ages lie down, to cover this false promise on rusting buckles: 'Gott Mit Uns.'" —Joe Haan, Alsace-Lorraine, France, 1944

"Here I was thousands of miles from home on foreign soil, sharing this hole with a dead man, this creature I had been indoctrinated to hate. Somehow, I had never quite pictured the enemy as totally human. Gradually it became clear to me that here was a victim of circumstance like myself." —Joe Haan, Alsace-Lorraine, France, 1944, sharing a foxhole with a German corpse

"Soldier's Lament—A violent thing I do today, in futile battle men I slay, who have been short years and a day, in time that here they had to stay." —Joe Haan, Alsace-Lorraine, France, 1944

"Those that I fight, I do not hate, those that I guard, I do not love. No likely end could bring me less, or leave me happier than before." —Joe Haan, Alsace-Lorraine, France, 1944

"Like a speeding locomotive that comes rushing down the track, you hear Eighty-Eight's a whistling just before you hear 'em crack." —Joe Haan, Alsace-Lorraine, France, 1944

"I owe one apology only, and that is to the devil, for lacking the ability to be more severe in my criticism of all organized religion." —Joe Haan, Houston, Texas, 1980

"If you read between the lines of my work, and not misinterpret it, you *will detect sheer unadulterated skepticism and also criticism to expose the mad vanity of all religion, the basic cause of war that served no ultimate purpose."* —Joe Haan, Houston, Texas, 1990

"For you can now see, as long as my birth, gods have not trod upon this earth." —Joe Haan, Houston, Texas, 1974

"My advice for the next generation—when all else fails, try common sense." —Joe Haan, Houston, Texas, 1974

"The finality of death is a terrible shock to the human ego, for we never pass this way again, a message constantly transmitted to us at every conscious moment of existence." —Joe Haan, Houston, Texas, 1980

"Only the lowly atom will survive without dissolution. Atoms without emotions, reason, personality, consciousness, or sentimentality; for the atom alone is godly—the reason for everything that exists—for even if god existed, that god would be as emotionless as the atom." —Joe Haan, Houston, Texas, 1980

"So, what fools we mortals be, to be snared in a heavenly sea. Do not take that scripture bait, avoid a boring, endless fate." —Joe Haan, Houston, Texas, 1974

"The cosmic shooting gallery of life." —Joe Haan, Houston, Texas, 1974

"Fido's Fate—Backward spell the word of Dog, you also have the word called God!" —Joe Haan, Houston, Texas, 1980

"Over this enigma of life and sudden violent death, for how does one reason out, this wasting of human intellect, the squandering of one who showed so much potential for further achievement in any field?" —Joe Haan, Houston, Texas, 1980

"In all the world of adventurous men, the high steel boy is one of them.

On gird or truss or bridging high, many a hand has had to die. —Joe Haan, Houston, Texas, 1980

"There are those who might say—they don't deserve that big iron pay. So come all you who speak as such, let's see if you dare to do as much."
—Joe Haan, Houston, Texas, 1980

"On Houston's Landor Lane lives the only white man in a sea of black."
—Joe Haan, Houston, Texas, 1980

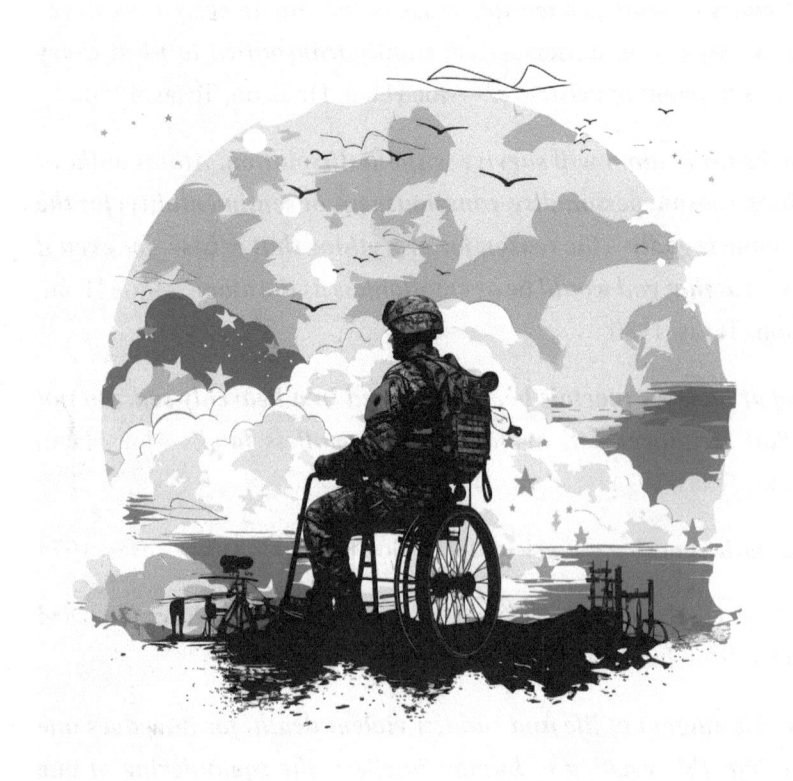

DIAL 988 —

TO BE EMPOWERED, THE DOC SAYS...

"FOR EVERYTHING THERE IS A SEASON…

A TIME TO BE BORN, AND A TIME TO DIE…

A TIME TO KILL AND A TIME TO HEAL…

A TIME TO BREAK DOWN, AND A TIME TO BUILD UP…

A TIME TO WEEP, AND A TIME TO LAUGH…

A TIME TO MOURN, AND A TIME TO DANCE…

A TIME FOR WAR, AND A TIME FOR PEACE."

ECCLESIASTES 3:1

Veterans in Crisis

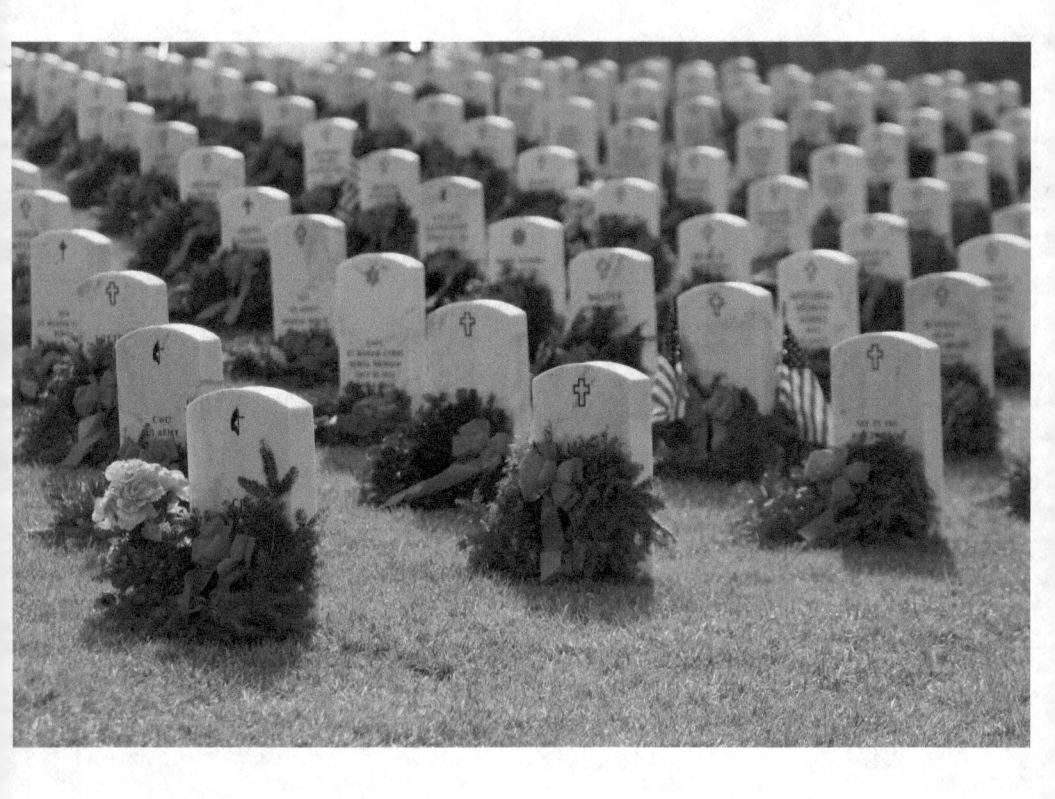

ACKNOWLEDGEMENTS

This book is a collection of true stories and writings about PTSD and its ancient history, published for medical and educational purposes to be given away free to suffering veterans and caregivers in VA and military hospitals, jails, prisons, veterans' organizations, and the like around America and where trauma severely affects people, as in our recent wars and in Ukraine today.

We have endeavored to seek written permission of copyright holders in advance when using materials or images that may not be in the public domain. We have the utmost respect for writers, photographers, podcasters, and film makers for material included in this book, and if for some reason we have used words or images without sufficiently due credit, please let us know.

We especially thank Dr. Bessel van der Kolk, M.D. and Penguin Books for the exceptional materials in the landmark book, *"The Body Keeps the Score,"* that we have quoted in Part II. It is considered a PTSD *"bible."*

We wish to thank Abigail Taylor, publication manager, for her professionalism in managing the intricacies of going from manuscript to publication; and Anna Weir, research assistant, for her invaluable work in tracking down several hundred images and illustrations. And Aaron Ferguson, whose talent designing the front and back covers of this book is equaled only by his talent in landscape design. A special thanks to Samantha Herr for the creation, design, and maintenance of our website www.vetsempowered.org.

Lake City, Rochester, Red Wing, and Wabasha colleagues and friends provided inspiration and unwavering support at critical times: Pete and Yvette Quist, Steve and Ann Lansing, Cliff and Annette Reynolds and Natalie Rose, Dori Lindsay, Steve and Tyler, Jennifer Shumaker, Jeremy Nelson, Tom Braun, Judge Joseph Chase of the Rochester Veterans Court, Frederico "Ever-Ready Freddy" Hernandez-Mozqueda, Tony Baloney, Wabasha County Sherriff Sergeant Mike Timm, a rap poet from Chicago, Red Wing Marine Corps League, Lake City VFW, and many Lake City friends and neighbors.

We owe the deepest appreciation to Cliff and Annette for their daily assistance and constant care; to Jeremy, Dori and Jenifer's PTSD group for their patience, acceptance, honesty, friendship, and everlasting support.

To our FUBAR Band of Brothers, fiercely independent mavericks molded at St. Olaf College in the 1950s in search of meaning, truth, and new adventure while embracing the existential and transcending traditional human behavior—thank you Fubars for the precious memories of our many times together while traveling the world in our many separate ways.

To Pete Quist, a special tribute for his resiliency and courage. Pete was able to hang in there with the Colonel through thick and thin, moving around the world and around the States. Sports and Pete's dynamic personality kept him connected and grounded with friends at each new duty station—from Olympia, WA where he was born, to Germany, Washington DC, Oklahoma, Colorado, Virginia, California, and finally back home in Minnesota.

Most of all, we owe appreciation and support for the millions of those who have served our nation, a mere 5% of the population. Those individuals were willing to raise their hand, take an oath, and serve their country so that the rest of us could be free. In their service, they were willing to undergo things that necessitate the writing of this book.

Our deepest recognition for those who have served, not just on the designated "special" days of the year but on each and every day of the year.

Acknowledgements

Without you, we would not have been able to write this book, and those reading these words would not be able to be present to continue on. To all past, present, and future warriors—You "dun" good.

A sincere and heartfelt thanks to all of you—Semper Fi, Anchors Away, to the Stars and Beyond—the Caissons keep rollin' along.

All the best,

Steve and Wayne

ARTICLES OF INCORPORATION & BYLAWS

Veterans Empowered Inc., A 501(c)3 Nonprofit

The undersigned, for the purpose of forming a nonprofit corporation under Chapter 317A of the laws of the State of Minnesota, does hereby make and adopt the following Articles of Incorporation:

ARTICLE I. The name of the corporation is: VETERANS EMPOWERED, INC.

ARTICLE II. The Mission of Veterans Empowered is to inform, assist, and convey information to U.S. Veterans suffering from traumatic stress and Post-Traumatic Stress Disorder (PTSD). Veterans Empowered Inc. is a Minnesota based nonprofit corporation formed to educate the population and raise funding for the purpose of counseling, collecting data, writing, publishing, and distributing PTSD materials free of charge to U.S. Veterans, hospitals, and organizations throughout the United States. A secondary purpose is to increase awareness for the general public as to the nature of military trauma and its long-term impact on those who have served. This increased awareness will serve to provide support and decrease the stigma both individually and collectively to those who suffer from PTSD and other trauma-related conditions.

ARTICLE III. The corporation does not afford pecuniary gain, incidentally or otherwise, to its members.

ARTICLE IV. The duration of the corporation is perpetual.

ARTICLE V. The corporation will seek tax exempt recognition under Section 501(c)(3) of the Internal Revenue Service Code.

ARTICLE VI. The corporation and its members shall not undertake any activity that may be prohibited by the Internal Revenue Service for organizations seeking tax exempt status.

ARTICLE VII. The location of the registered office of this corporation within the State of Minnesota is: 117 East Center Street, Rochester, MN 55904.

ARTICLE VIII. The name and post office address of the incorporator of this corporation is as follows: Thomas R. Braun, 117 East Center Street, Rochester, MN 55904.

ARTICLE IX. Four directors shall constitute the first Board of Directors, and they shall serve until the first annual meeting of the corporation or until their successors are sooner or thereafter duly elected and qualified, and their names and respective addresses are as follows:

Thomas Braun, Director & Board Chair (Attorney).

Steven Lansing, Director & President (U.S. Air Force, Vietnam Veteran).

Cliff Reynolds, Director & Vice President (U.S. Army, Vietnam Veteran).

Jon Peters, Director and Vice President, U.S. Navy Corpsman (USMC), Vietnam Veteran.

B. Wayne Quist, Director & Secretary/Treasurer (USMC/USAF Vietnam/ME Veteran).

Jeremy Nelson, Director (U.S. Army Green Beret, Afghanistan/Special Ops Veteran).

Ann Lansing, Director (Certified Addictions Registered Nurse).

Coltin Schmidt, Director (Probation Officer, Veterans Court).

Jennifer Schumaker, Director (U.S. Army Afghanistan Veteran, V.S.O.).

Preston Selleck, Director (U.S. Marine Corps Afghanistan Veteran, Attorney).

Christine Lueders, Director (Paralegal).

Dan Ludwig, Director, Veteran U.S. Navy Nuclear Submarine Service, Past State and National Commander American Legion.

Dori, Lindsay, Director & Events Coordinator, Retired History Teacher.

Lance Garrick, Director, Veteran, U.S. Army retired, Commander Red Wing MN American Legion.

Danny Bucknell, Director Bank Vice President

ARTICLE X. There shall be no personal liabilities of the members of the corporation for corporate obligations.

ARTICLE XI. This corporation is organized on a non-stock basis. This corporation shall not issue shares of stock.

ARTICLE XII. Upon the dissolution of the corporation, assets shall be distributed for one or more exempt purposes within the meaning of section 501(c)(3) of the Internal Revenue Code or the corresponding section of any future Federal tax code. Any assets not so disposed shall be disposed of by a court of competent jurisdiction of the county in which the principal office of the corporation is located. Disposal shall be made exclusively for exempt or public purposes or be made to such organization or organizations as the court shall determine to be organized exclusively for such purposes.

BY-LAWS OF VETERANS EMPOWERED, INC.

ARTICLE I. Corporate Powers

In furtherance of the express purposes of this corporation, all as are more fully set forth in the Articles of Incorporation, the corporation shall have, and exercise, all the powers conferred upon it by the statutes of the State of Minnesota, now existing or as hereinafter amended or enacted.

ARTICLE II. Corporate Purpose

Section 1. Nonprofit Purpose. This corporation is organized exclusively for charitable, religious, counseling, educational, and scientific purposes, including, for such purposes, the making of distributions to organizations that qualify as exempt organizations under section 501(c)(3) of the Internal Revenue Code or the corresponding section of any future federal tax code.

Section 2. Specific Purpose. The purpose of the corporation is to educate, inform, assist, counsel, and convey information to U.S. Veterans suffering from traumatic stress and Post-Traumatic Stress Disorder (PTSD). Veterans Empowered Inc. is a Minnesota-based nonprofit corporation formed to educate the population and raise funding for the purpose of collecting data, writing, publishing, and distributing written PTSD materials free of charge to U.S. Veterans, hospitals, and organizations throughout the United States. A secondary purpose is to increase awareness of the general public as to the nature of military trauma and its long-term on those who have served. This increased awareness will serve to provide support and decrease the stigma both individually and collectively to those who suffer from PTSD and other trauma related conditions.

ARTICLE III. Board of Directors

Section 1 - General Powers. The affairs of the corporation shall be managed by its Board of Directors, which shall have the power to transact all business of the corporation in accordance with these Bylaws and the provisions of the Minnesota Nonprofit Corporation Act, Minnesota Statutes 317.A, and all future laws amendatory thereof and supplementary thereto, not inconsistent with these Bylaws and the Articles of Incorporation.

Section 2 Number, Tenure and Qualifications. The Board of Directors of the corporation shall consist of at least three (3), but not more than ten (10), members. Once elected, a director serves for an indefinite term that expires at the next regular meeting of the corporation. A director holds office for the term for which the director was elected and until a successor is elected by a majority vote of the members of the Board of Directors and has qualified, or until the director's earlier death, resignation, removal, or disqualification. The name and address of each member of the first Board of Directors shall be those persons identified in the Articles of Incorporation. The term of office of each such member of the first Board of Directors shall be until such Director's successor shall have been appointed or selected or shall otherwise qualify for office.

Section 3 Annual Meeting. The Board of Directors shall conduct its annual meeting on the day or date, and at the time and place, as shall be fixed by a resolution adopted by a majority of the Directors.

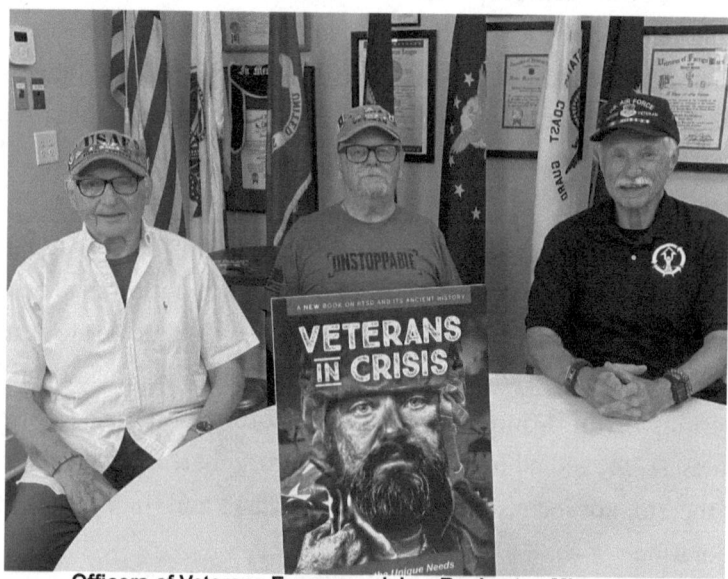

Officers of Veterans Empowered, Inc. Rochester, Minnesota.
(L-R) Colonel B. Wayne Quist Secretary/Treasurer; Sp5 Cliff Reynolds, Vice President, Sgt. Dr. Steve Lansing, President

Section 4 Regular Meetings. Regular meetings of the Board of Directors shall be held on the day or date, and at the time and place, as may from time to time be fixed by resolution adopted by a majority of the Directors.

Veterans Empowered, Inc.
Rochester, Minnesota
Mission Big Willy-Won

SOURCES & REFERENCES

- 752nd Field Artillery Battalion. History, Verdun, France, 15 August 1945. Unpublished unit history, Joe Haan poems and notebooks in author's collection, Millersburg Schoolhouse Museum, Millersburg, MN.
- Adams, Michael C. "Living Hell: The Dark Side of the Civil War." Johns Hopkins University Press, Baltimore, 2014.
- Allison, Graham, "Destined for War: Can America and China Escape Thucydides Trap?" Mariner Books, 2017.
- Amar, Akhil Reed. "The Words That Made US: America's Constitutional Conversation, 1760-1840." Basic Books, 2021.
- Ambrose, Stephen. "Band of Brothers." Simon & Schuster, 2001.
- Ambrose, Stephen. "Citizen Soldiers." Simon & Schuster, 1997.
- Ambrose, Stephen. "D-Day June 6, 1944: The Climactic Battle of WWII." Simon & Schuster, 1995.
- Ambrose, Stephen. "The Victors: Eisenhower and His Boys: The Men of World War II." Simon & Schuster, 1998.
- Ambrose, Stephen. "The Wild Blue: The Men and Boys Who Flew the B-24s Over Germany 1944-45." Simon & Schuster, 2001.
- Andrew P., MD. "The Alcoholic/Addict Within: Our Brain, Genetics, Psychology and the Twelve Steps as Psychotherapy." Amazon e-Book. 2017.
- Appel and Beebe, "Preventive Psychiatry," Journal of AMA (1946).
- Atkinson, Rick. "Guns at First Light: The War in Western Europe, 1944-1945." Henry Holt and Company, 2013.
- Atkinson, Rick. "The Day of battle: The War in Sicily and Italy, 1943-1944." Henry Holt and Company, 2007.
- Bagnall, S. "The Attack," London: Hamish, 1947.
- Barker, Kenneth, General Ed. "The NIV Study Bible." Zondervan Bible Publishers, 1985.
- Barker, Pat. "Regeneration." Plume, Penguin Random, 1992.
- Bartone, Paul T. et al, eds. "Applying Army Research Psychology for Health and Performance Gains." Technology and National Security Policy, National Defense University, Washington, D.C. August 2010.

- Bentley, Steve. "A short history of PTSD." VVA Veteran, Silver Spring, MD. 2005.
- Bierce, Ambrose. "The Devil's Dictionary." The Library of America.
- Billings, John D. "Hardtack and Coffee or The Unwritten Story of Army Life." Boston, George M. Smith and Company, 1888.
- Bradley, John R. "Saudi Arabia Exposed: Inside a Kingdom in Crisis." Palgrave MacMillan, 2005.
- Brands, Hal, ed. "The New Makers of Modern Strategy: From the Ancient World to the Digital Age." Princeton University Press, 2023.
- Braundel, Fernand. "A History of Civilizations." Penguin, 1994.
- Bremner, J.Douglas. Invisible Epidemic: Post-Traumatic stress Disorder, Memory and the Brain." Pandora's Project 2001-2009.
- Burroughs, John. "Notes on Walt Whitman, As Poet and Person." Second Edition. J.S. Redfield, New York, 1871.
- Caesar, Julius. "War Commentaries." Rex Warner (tr), 1960.
- Caplan, Fred. "Wizards of Armageddon." Simon and Schuster, 1983.
- Caputo, Philip. "A Rumor of War." Ballantine Books, NY 1977.
- Catton, Bruce. "Grant Moves South," Doubleday & Co. NY: 1963 (Volume III of The Centennial History of the Civil War, 3 volumes).
- Catton, Bruce. "Mr. Lincoln's Army." Anchor Books, September 1990.
- Catton, Bruce. "Terrible Swift Sword," Doubleday & Co. NY: 1963 (Volume II of The Centennial History of the Civil War, 3 volumes).
- Catton, Bruce. "The Coming Fury," Doubleday & Co. NY: 1963 (Volume I of The Centennial History of the Civil War, 3 volumes).
- Chesnut, Mary Boykin. Williams, Ben Ames, ed. "A Diary From Dixie." Houghton Mifflin Company, Boston. 1905, 1949.
- Christy, Annette; Clark, Colleen; Frei, Autumn; and Rynearson-Moody Sarah. "Challenges of Diverting Veterans to Trauma Informed Care: The Heterogeneity of Intercept 2." Criminal Justice and Behavior, 2012 39: 461. Published online 14 February 2012.
- Cicero, Marcus Tullius. "Selected Political Speeches." Michael Grant. (tr) 1977.

- Clarke, Daniel. MA Thesis: "Post-Traumatic Stress Disorder and the American Civil War: A Reappraisal." Academia.edu. Accessed 4-23-2022. https://www.academia.edu/5812575/Post_Traumatic_Stress_Disorder_and_the_American_Civil_War_A_Reappraisal.
- Clement, Priscilla Ferguson. "With Wise and Benevolent Purpose: Poor Children and the State Public School at Owatonna, 1885—1915." Minnesota History (Spring 1984). http://collections.mnhs.org/MNHistoryMagazine/articles/49/v49i01p002-013.pdf (accessed August 2023).
- Congressional Research Service. "American War and Military Operations, Casualties: Lists and Statistics." RL32492. July 29, 2020.
- Conroy, Pat. "The Great Santini." Dial Press, NY, 2013.
- Courtwright, David. "Opiate Addiction as a Consequence of the Civil War." Civil War History 24, 1978.
- Crane, Hart. "The Bridge. "Liveright Publishing, NY, London, 1933, 1958, 1970.
- Creech, Suzannah K. and Misca, Gabriela. "Parenting with PTSD: A Review of Research on the Influence of PTSD on Parent-Child Functioning in Military and Veteran Families." Frontiers in Psychology. 30 June 2017, p 1-8. https://doi.org/10.3389/fpsyg.2017.01101
- Crocq, Marc-Antoine MD and Crocq, Louis MD. "From shell shock and war neurosis to posttraumatic stress disorder: a history of psychotraumatology." Dialogues in Clinical Neuroscience, Volume 2, page 47-55, 1 April 2022.
- Cross, Wilbur and Brooke, Tucker, eds. "The Tragedy of Macbeth." The Yale Shakespeare: The Complete Works. Barnes and Noble Books, New York, 1993.
- Cross, Wilbur L. and Brooke, Tucker, eds. "The Yale Shakespeare Complete Works." Barnes and Noble, 1993.
- Da Costa, J. M. (1871). "On irritable heart; A clinical study of a form of functional cardiac disorder and its consequences." American Journal of the Medical Sciences, 121(1).
- Davis, Washington. "Camp-Fire Chats." Grand Army of the Republic (GAR), 1884. Big Byte Books, 2014.
- Dean, Eric T. Jr. "We Will All Be Lost And Destroyed: Post-Traumatic Stress Disorder and the Civil War." Civil War History. The Kent State University Press, Volume 37, Number 2, June 1991.

Sources & References

- Dean, Eric T. Jr. "Shook Over Hell: Post-Traumatic Stress, Vietnam, and the Civil War." Harvard University Press, Cambridge MA, London, 1997.
- Department of Defense, Defense Health agency, Psychological Health Center of Excellence, Psychological Health Readiness, Combat and Operational Stress Control (COSC), Combat and Operational Stress Reactions (COSRs).
- Dilberger, J. Thomas. Book # 873894, Local 361 (Retiree). "Blacks and High Steel: What affirmative action did to the trade." The Ironworker, June 2006.
- District of Columbia Department of Mental Health (n.d.). "St. Elizabeth's Hospital's expanded role during the Civil War." http://dmh.dc.gov/dmh/cwp/view,a,3,q,636030.asp
- Doerries, Bryan. "The Theater of War." Vintage Books, 2015.
- Douds, Anne S.; Ahlin, Eileen M.; Howard, Daniel, and Stigerwalt, Sarah. "Varieties of Veterans' Courts: A Statewide Assessment of Veterans' Treatment Court Components." Criminal Justice Policy Review, 2017, Vol. 28(8).
- Dupuy, Colonel R. Ernest and Dupuy, Colonel Trevor N., USA (Ret). The Encyclopedia of Military History." Harper & Row, NY 1970.
- Durant, Will and Ariel, "The Story of Civilization," eleven volumes. Simon and Schuster, 1939.
- Dyer, Gwynne. "War." Crown Publishers Inc., NY, 1985. Periscope, UK, 2017.
- Egger, Bruce and Otts, Leo MacMillan. "G Company's War: Two Personal Accounts of the Campaigns in Europe, 1944-1945. The University of Alabama Press, 1992.
- European Journal of Psychtraumatology. 2019.
- Fix, Lianna; Kimmage, Michael; Kagan, Robert; Zugart, Amy. "The World Putin Made." Foreign Affairs, January/February 2023.
- Folger Shakespeare Theater. "Advice from the players: 10 great actors on performing Shakespeare." July 21, 2023. https://www.folger.edu
- Friedman, Matthew J. MD. "'Soldier's heart' and 'shell shock': Past names for PTSD." Department of Veterans Affairs, 2005. http://www.pbs.org/wgbh/pages/frontline/shows/heart/themes/shellshock.html
- Fussell, Paul. "The Great War and Modern Memory." Oxford University Press, 1977.
- Fussell, Paul. "Wartime: Understanding and Behavior in the Second World War." Oxford: Oxford University Press, 1989.

- Gabriel, Richard A. "No More Heroes." Prime 1987.
- Garwath, Robert. "The Vanquished: Why the First World War Failed to End." Farrar, Straus & Giroux, 2016.
- Gordon, John B. Major General, Confederate Army. "Reminiscences of the Civil War." Charles Scribner's Sons, 1904, 2018.
- Graves, Robert. "Good-Bye To All That." Random House, 1929, 1957, 1985, 1989, 1998.
- Gray, J. Glenn. "The Warriors: Reflections on Men in Battle." University of Nebraska Press, Lincoln and London, 1959.
- Grinker, Roy R. "War Neuroses in North Africa: The Tunisian Campaign, January-May 1943." University of California Libraries reprint.
- Grinker, Roy R. Lt. Col. and Spiegel, John P. Major. "Men Under Stress." Army Air Forces (AAF) Convalescent Hospital, St. Petersburg, FL. 1945. Pickle Partners Publishing, 2017.
- Grossman, Dave, Army Ranger and Military Historian. "On Killing." Little Brown and Company, 2009.
- Grossman, Dave, Army Ranger and Military Historian; and Davis, Adam. "On Spiritual Combat: 30 Missions for Victorious Combat." Broadstreet Publishing. 2020.
- Guanzhong, Luo. "The Romance of Three Kingdoms." Penguin, 2018.
- Haahr, James C., "The Command is Forward: The 101st Infantry in Lorraine," Xlibris, 2003.
- Haan Family Records. Files #7993, #7994, #7995. Minnesota History Center. Minnesota State Historical Society Archives. Owatonna State School Records. St. Paul, Minnesota.
- Haan, Joe. Unpublished Army records, poems, and notebooks, BW Quist collection; Millersburg Schoolhouse Museum, Millersburg, Minnesota.
- Haapoja, Margaret A. "Back to Work." Forest Magazine, Summer 2009. https://www.fseee.org/about-us/ (accessed August 2023).
- Hamel, Debra. "Socrates at War: The Military Heroics of an Iconic Intellectual." Kindle Edition, 2013. Revised version of article originally published in MHQ: The Quarterly Journal of Military History.
- Hastings, Donald, Major, et al. "Psychiatric Experience of the Eighth Air Force First Year of Combat June 1942 to June 1943." U.S. Army Air Force, Air Surgeon, 1944.

- Hay, John, Lt. Gen. "Vietnam Studies." Washington: Department of the Army, 1974.
- Hemingway, Ernest. "A Farewell to Arms." Scribner, New York, 1929, 1957, 2012.
- Herken, Gregg. "Counsels of War." Knopf, 1985.
- Herodotus. "The Histories." Penguin 1951.
- History of PTSD. https://historyofptsd.wordpress.com/early-history/
- Holmes, Lee. "Lucretius–On the Nature of Things." Atheist Foundation of Australia, Inc. https://atheistfoundation.org.au/ (accessed August 2023).
- Holt, Dean. "American Military Cemeteries: A Comprehensive Illustrated Guide to the Hallowed Grounds of the United States, Including Cemeteries Overseas." Jefferson, NC: McFarland & Co., 1992.
- Homer, "Iliad." University of Chicago Press, 1951.
- Homer, "Odyssey." University of Chicago Press, 1951.
- Horvath, Edward P. M.D. "Good Medicine, Hard Times: A Memoir of a Combat Physician in Iraq." The Ohio State University, 2022."
- Horwitz, Tony. "Did Civil War Soldiers Have PTSD?" Smithsonian Magazine. Jan 2015. https://www.smithsonianmag.com/history/ptsd-civil-wars-hidden-legacy-180953652/
- Huntington, Samuel. "The Clash of Civilizations: Remaking of World Order." Simon and Schuster, 1996.
- Huntington, Samuel. "The Soldier and the State," NY: Vintage 1964.
- Huskey, Kristine A. "Reconceptualizing 'the Crime in Veterans Treatment Courts." Federal Sentencing Reporter, vol. 27, no. 3. February 2015.
- Ingersoll, Robert Green. "Great Speeches of Colonel R. G. Ingersoll." Chicago: Rhodes & McClure, 1895.
- Johnson, Rossiter. "Martial Epitaphs." The Century, a Popular Quarterly Vol. 40, No.1 (May 1890).
- Joshi, S.T. "Ambrose Bierce: The Devil's Dictionary, Tales, & Memoirs." The Library of America, New York, 2011.
- Kagan, Donald. "Pericles of Athens and the Birth of Democracy." The Free Press, 1991.
- Kagan, Donald. "The Peloponnesian War." Penguin, 2003.

- Kane, Shawn F. MD; Saperstein, Adam K. MD; Bunt, Christopher W. MD; Stephens, Mark B. MD. "When War Follows Combat Veterans Home." Department of Family Medicine, Uniformed Services University of the Health Sciences, Bethesda, MD. The Journal of Family Practice, vol. 62, no. 8, August 2013.

- Kaplan, Robert D. "Marco Polo's World: War, Strategy and American Interests in the Twenty-First Century." Random House, 2018.

- Kardiner, Abram and Spiegel, Herbert. "War Stress and Neurotic Illness." Medical Book Department of Harper and Brothers, New York, London,1947.

- Kardiner, Abram. "The Traumatic Neuroses of War." Martino Publishing, Medical Book Department of Harper and Brothers, New York, London 1941.

- Keagan, John. "A History of Warfare." Alfred A. Knopf, 1993.

- Keagan, John. "Face of Battle." NY: Penguin Books 1978.

- Keagan, John. "The First World War." Alfred A. Knopf, 1998.

- Keeling, Arlene, PhD, RN. "The Nurses of Mayo Clinic." Mayo Foundation, 2014.

- Keith, Gabe (USMC). "Little Warrior Brother." Self-Published, 2017.

- Kennedy, David M., editor. "The Library of Congress World War II Companion." New York, Simon & Schuster 2007.

- Kennedy, Hugh. "The Great Arab Conquests." Da Capo Press, 2009.

- Kennedy. Kelly. "They Fought for Each Other: The Triumph and Tragedy of the Hardest Hit Unit in Iraq." St. Martin's Griffin, 2011.

- Kissinger, Henry. "Diplomacy." Simon and Schuster, 1994.

- Kissinger, Henry. "On China." Penguin, 2012.

- Kissinger, Henry. "World Order." Penguin, 2014.

- Klein, Sara. "The Three Major Stress Hormones, Explained." Huffington Post, April 19, 2013.

- Krenzel, Robert. "Quill and Ink: Post Traumatic Stress in the American Revolution." https://www.amazon.com/Times-That-Try-Mens-Souls/dp/1635030420/

- Kushner, Harold S. "When Bad Things Happen to Good People." Random House 1981.

- Kussmaul, Allen. "Life on the Bum in the Early 1930s." AuthorHouse, 2009.
- Lacey, Robert. "Inside the Kingdom." Penguin, 2009.
- Lacey, Robert. "The Kingdom: Arabia & The House of Sa'ud." Blackstone Publishing, 2018.
- Lande, R. Gregory. "Madness, Malingering & Malfeasance." Brassey's Inc. Washington, DC. 2003.
- Leinbaugh, Harold P. and Campbell, John D. "The Men of Company K: The Autobiography of a World War II Rifle Company." Bantam, 1987.
- LeShan, Lawrence. "The Psychology of War." New York: Helios Press, 2002.
- Lewis, Ralph, MD. "Finding Purpose in a Godless World." Prometheus Books, 2018.
- Linder, Douglas. "Clarence Seward Darrow, 1857-1938." University of Missouri-Kansas City (UMKC) School of Law.
- Linderman, Gerald F. "Embattled Courage: The Experience of Combat in the American Civil War." Macmillan, Inc., New York, 1987.
- Livy, Titus. "History of Rome." 4 volumes, various translators, Penguin 1965-1982.
- Logue, Larry M. "To Appomattox and Beyond: The Civil War Soldier in War and Peace." The American Way Series. Ivan R. Dee, Chicago, 1996.
- Logue, Larry M. and Barton, Michael, eds. "The Civil War Veteran: A Historical Reader." New York University Press, 2007.
- Lounsbury, Thomas R., ed. Yale Book of American Verse. 1912. http://bartleby.com/102/147.html (accessed August 2023).
- Lucado, Max. "You'll Get Through This." Thomas Nelson, 2013.
- MacDonald, Charles B. "The Last Offensive" (United States Army in World War II: The European Theater of Operations). Konecky & Konecky, 1973.
- MacMillan, Margaret. "Paris 1919: Six Months That Changed the World." Random House, 2003.
- MacMillan, Margaret. "The War That Ended Peace: The Road to 1914." Random House, 2013.
- MacMillan, Margaret. "War: How Conflict Shaped Us." Random House, 2020.
- Mahedy, William P. "Out of he Night: The Spiritual Journey of Vietnam Vets." Radix Press, 2004.

- Marlantes, Karl. "What it's Like to go to War." NY: Atlantic Monthly Press, 2011.
- Marshall, S.L.A., "Men Against Fire." 1947, University of Texas El Paso, S.L.A. Marshal Military history Collection.
- McPherson, James M. "Battle Cry of Freedom." Oxford University Press, 1988.
- Miller, Donald A. "Masters of the Air: America's Bomber Boys Who Fought the Air War Against Nazi Germany." Simon and Schuster, New York, London, 2006.
- Monoson, S. Sara. "Combat Trauma and The Ancient Greeks: Socrates In Combat." New York 2014.
- Monroe, Robert A. "Journeys Out of the Body." Harmony Books, New York, 1971.
- Moran, Lord Captain Charles Wilson. "The Anatomy of Courage: The Classical World War I Account of the Psychological Effects of War." Carroll & Graf Publishers, New York, 1945, 2007.
- Murawiec, Laurent. "Princes of Darkness: The Saudi Assault on the West." Trans. by George Holoch. Rowman & Littlefield, 2003.
- Musgrave, John. "Notes to the Man Who Shot Me: Vietnam War Poems." Self-Published, 2003.
- National Museum of Civil War Medicine, "Post Traumatic Stress Disorder and the American Civil War." May 2, 2019.
- Ninh, Bao. "The Sorrow of War: A Novel of North Vietnam." Anchor Books, 2018.
- NOVA, "Your Brain: Perception Deception Neuroscientists discover the tricks and shortcuts the brain takes to help us survive." PBS NOVA. May 17, 2003. https://www.pbs.org/wgbh/nova/video/your-brain-perception-deception/
- O'Brien, Tim. "The Things They Carried." Mariner Books, 2009.
- O'Hara, Theodore. "Bivouac of the Dead." Department of Veteran Affairs, March 2009. http://www.cem.va.gov/hist/BODpoem.asp
- Office of the Quartermaster General. "Annual Reports of the War Department, 1822-1907." National Archives and Records Administration. RG 92, Microfilm (M997).

Sources & References

- Office of the Quartermaster General. "Roll of Honor." 25 vols. Washington, DC: Government Printing Office, 1868-71. Baltimore: Genealogical Publishing Co., 1994.
- Offley, Ed. "Norman Schwarzkopf." Seattle Post Intelligencer October 6, 1992.
- Packer, George. "The Assassin's Gate: America in Iraq." Farrar, Straus and Giroux, NY, 2005.
- Pierce, Andrew G., MCAP. "Resolving Spiritual Skepticism in Recovery." O'Leary Publishing, 2023.
- Pillsbury, Michael. "The Hundred-Year Marathon: China's Secret Strategy to Replace America as the Global Superpower." Henry Holt and Co., 2015.
- Poe, Edgar Allan. "Sixty-Seven Tales, One Complete Novel and Thirty-One Poems." Amaranth, 1985.
- Polo, Marco, "The Travels of Marco Polo, the Venetian." Trans. W. Marsden and newly revised by Peter Harris. Everyman's Library, 1908, 2008.
- Polybius, "The Rise of the Roman Empire." Ian Scott-Kilvert (tr) 1979.
- Qiao, Liang, Colonel and Xiangsui Wang, Colonel. "Unrestricted Warfare." People's Liberation Army, China, 1999.
- Quist, B. Wayne. "God's Angry Man: The Incredible Journey of Private Joe Haan." Brown Books, Dallas, 2010.
- Rasenberger, Jim. "High Steel: The Daring Men Who Built the World's Greatest Skyline." New York, NY: HarperCollins Publishers, Inc., 2004.
- Remarque, Erich Maria. "Eight Stories: Tales of War and Loss." Washington Mews Books, NY, 2028.
- Resnick, P.A.; Monson, C.M. & Chard, K.M. "Cognitive Processing Therapy: Veteran/Military Version Therapist's Manual." Department of Veterans' Affairs, National Center for PTSD, 2008.
- Ricks, Tom. "Fiasco: The American Military Adventure in Iraq." Penguin. 2006.
- Ricks, Tom. "The Gamble: General David Petraeus and the American Military Adventure in Iraq, 2006-2008." Penguin, 2009.
- Ricks, Tom. "The Generals: American Military Command from World War II to Today." Penguin, 2012.
- Rittenhouse, Jessie B., ed. "Little Book of American Poets: 1787-1900." Cambridge: Riverside Press, 1915.

- Rivers, W.H.R. "Instinct and the Unconscious." London: 1919. Appendix III, "Repression of War Experience."
- Rivers, W.H.R. "War Neurosis and Military Training" (1918).
- Ronglien, Harvey. "A Boy from C-11: Case #9164." Minnesota: Graham Megyeri Books, 2006.
- Ronglien, Harvey. Interviews with B. Wayne Quist, May, October, 2009.
- Rottman, Gordon L. "Fubar: Soldier Slang of World War II." Osprey Pub, 2007.
- Russell, Mark C.; Figley, Charles R. & Robertson, Kirsten R. "Investigating the Psychiatric Lessons of War and Pattern of Preventable Wartime Behavioral Health Crises." Journal of Psychology and Behavioral Science, Vol. 3, No. 1, pp. 1-12, June 2015.
- Sacks, Oliver. "Hallucinations." Vintage Books, 2013.
- Sallust, "Jugurthine War" ("Bellum Jugurthinum"). S.A. Handford (tr) 1963.
- Sanchelli, Michael T. "The Greatest Generation." Minnesota Historical Society, St. Paul, Minnesota, October 2006.
- Sassoon, Siegfried. "Sherston's Progress: The Memoirs of George Sherston." London: Penguin Books, 1936, 1964.
- Shay, Jonathan, M.D., PhD. "Achilles in Vietnam: Combat Trauma and the Undoing of Character." Scribner, 1994.
- Shay, Jonathan, M.D., PhD. "Odysseus in America." Scribner, 2002.
- Shephard, Ben. "A War of Nerves: Soldiers and Psychiatrists, 1914-1994." London, Jonathan Cape, 2000.
- Sholokov, Mikhail; Garry, Stephen translator. "And Quiet Flows the Don." Vintage International, 1989; Alfred A. Knopf, 1934, 1961.
- Skinner, P.M. and Kaplick, R. "Cultural shift in mental illness: a comparison of stress responses in World War I and the Vietnam War." December 2017. https://pubmed.ncbi.nlm.nih.gov/29230306/
- Smith, David A. "The Price of Valor: The Life of Audie Murphy." Regenery, 2016.
- Smithsonian Magazine. https://www.si.edu/newsdesk/photos?page=113
- Soodalter, Ron, "The Shock of War." May 2017 HistoryNet, Accessed April 23, 2022. https://www.historynet.com/the-shock-of-war/

Sources & References

- Sophocles. "Ajax," "Antigone," Oedipus Rex;" E-Bookarama Edition, Kindle 2021.
- Steinbeck, John. "Once There Was A War." Penguin Books, 1977.
- Stillman, Sarah. The New Yorker, "Hiroshima and the Inheritance of Trauma," August 12, 2014.
- Stouffer, et al. "The American Soldier," Vol. II, NJ: Princeton Univ. Press, 1949.
- Tanielian, Terri and Jaycox, Lisa H., eds. "Invisible Wounds of War: Psychological and Cognitive Injuries, Their Consequences, and Services to Assist Recovery." RAND Corporation, 2008.
- The Gale Encyclopedia of Medicine. Editor Ed Laurie J. Gale, Cengage 2011.
- The Gale Encyclopedia of Neurological Disorders. Second Edition. Editor Brigham Narins, Gale, Cengage Learning. 2012.
- Thucydides, "History of the Peloponnesian War." Penguin, 1954.
- Tick, Edward, PhD. "War and the Soul." Quest Books, 2005.
- Tick, Edward, PhD. "Warriors Return: Restoring the soul After War." Sounds True, 2014.
- Tolstoy, Leo. "War and Peace." Vintage Classics, 2008.
- Trittle, Lawrence A. "From Melos to My Lai." Routledge, NY, 2000.
- Tuchman, Barbara W. Alfred A. Knopf, NY 1984."The March of Folly: From Troy to Vietnam."
- U.S. Department of Justice Publication. "Defining Drug Courts: The Key Components." USGPO, Washington DC, 1997.
- Underwood, Doug. "Chronicling Trauma: Journalists and Writers on Violence and Loss." University of Illinois Press, Urbana, Chicago, 2011.
- United States National Library of Medicine (n.d.). Saint Elizabeth's Hospital. Retrieved August 2022 from http://www.nlm.nih.gov/hmd/medtour/elizabeths.html
- Van Der Kolk, Bessel. "The Body Keeps the Score: Brain, Mind and Body in the Healing of Trauma." Penguin Books, 2014.
- Vietnam Veterans of America: "The Veteran." Retrieved from http://www.vva.org/archive/TheVeteran/2005_03/feature_HistoryPTSD.htm

- Vonnegut, Kurt. "A Man Without A Country." Random House, Inc., NY, 2007.
- Vonnegut, Kurt. "Bluebeard." Random House, New York, 1987, 2011.
- Vonnegut, Kurt. "Cat's Cradle." Dial Press Trade 2010.
- Vonnegut, Kurt. "Slaughterhouse-Five." Random House, Inc., New York, 1969.
- Wells, Timothy S., et al. "Mental health impact of the Iraq and Afghanistan conflicts: A review of US research, service provision, and programmatic responses." American Psychiatry Review, April 2011.
- Wilson, A.N. "Tolstoy." Norton, 2001.
- Wilson, Jean Moorcroft. "Robert Graves: From Great War Poet to Good-bye to All That (1895-1929)." Bloomsbury Continuum, London, New York, 2018.
- Wilson, Robert Burns. "Theodore O'Hara." The Century, a Popular Quarterly, Vol. 40, No.1 (May 1890).
- Wounded Warrior Project. https://www.woundedwarriorproject.org/mission
- Yankee Division. "26th Infantry Division – World War II." http://yd-info.net/page2/index.html#Bulge (accessed August 2023).
- Zasiekina, Larysa, et al. "Post-traumatic Stress Disorder and Moral Injury Among Ukrainian Civilians During the Ongoing War." NIH National Library of Medicine. https://www.ncbi.nlm.nih.gov/pmc/articles/PMC10148618/

Sources & References

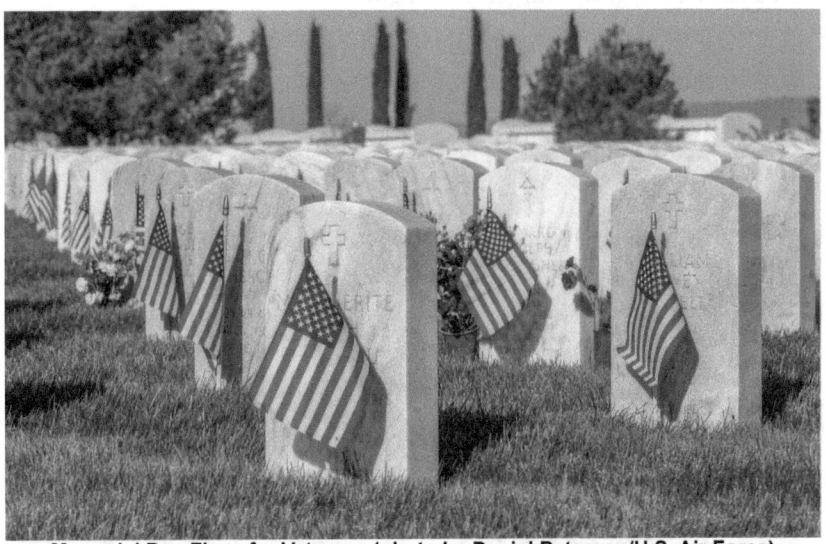

Memorial Day Flags for Veterans (photo by Daniel Peterson/U.S. Air Force)

Veterans in Crisis

U.S. ARMY SPC TONY HEBERT 1987-2007 KIA IRAQ

U.S. Army Sp-4 Tony Hebert, age 19, Lake City, Minnesota.

Killed in Action, Iraq "Surge," June 2007.

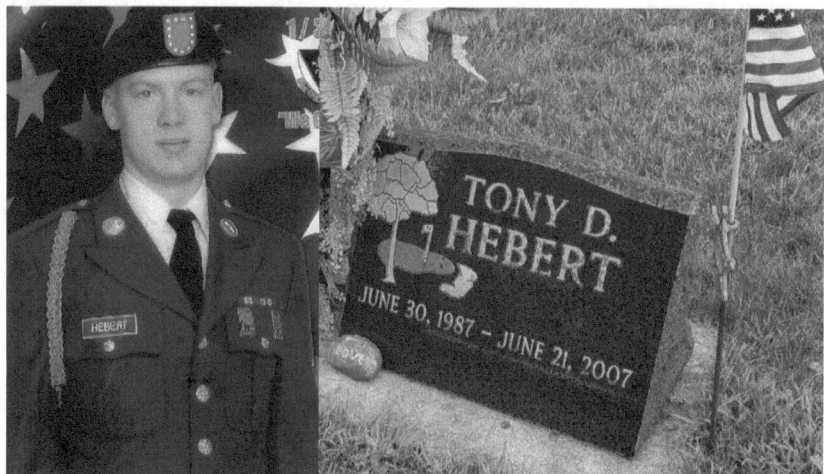

Photo (r) by Cliff Reynolds

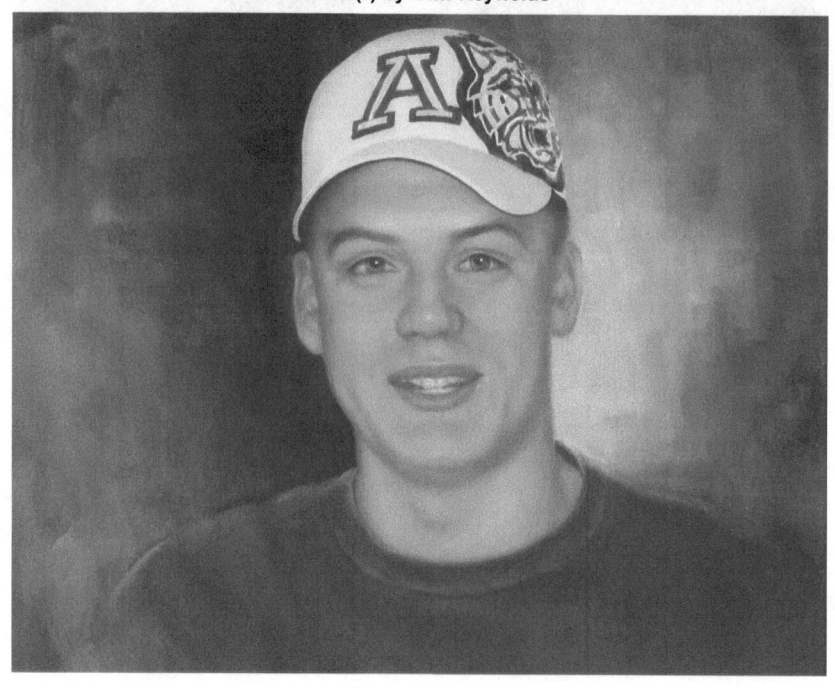

"Greater love hath no man than this, that a man lay down his life for his friends."

JOHN 15:13

"Honor to the Soldier, and Sailor everywhere, who bravely bears his country's cause ... for the common good, the storms of heaven and the storms of battle."

ABRAHAM LINCOLN, DECEMBER 2, 1863

> "Undermine your enemy, subvert him, sow discord among his leaders."
>
> **SUN TZU**
> *Chinese military general, strategist, philosopher, writer, author of "The Art of War," died 496 BC*

> "Wherever the art of medicine is loved, there is also a love of humanity."
>
> **HIPPOCRATES**
> *460–370 BC, "Father of Medicine"*

BGEN WILLIAM H. RUPERTUS, US MARINE CORPS, 1942

"Men must be made to understand "that the only weapon which stands between them and death is the rifle ... they must understand that their rifle is their life ... it must become a creed with them."

THE AUTHORS

The "Doc" – Steve Lansing, PhD, LICSW

- Vietnam veteran in country 1968–1970, active-duty U.S. Air Force 1966-1972.
- Licensed therapist specializing in trauma and PTSD with a focus on veterans and other victims of severe trauma.
- Mental health specialist, Minnesota Veteran's Treatment Court.
- In long-term recovery.
- Founder of dual recovery program – EmPower CTC, Rochester, Minnesota.
- President, Veterans Empowered, Inc., Rochester, Minnesota.

"The Colonel" – B. Wayne Quist, USAF Retired, private USMCR

- Vietnam veteran in country 1964–1968, Middle East 1968–1989.
- Advanced degrees in management, history, international relations, and psychology.
- Published author on war trauma, history, and international relations.
- In long-term recovery.
- Secretary/Treasurer, Veterans Empowered, Inc., Rochester, Minnesota.

MY JOURNEY – STEVE LANSING

Helping those with PTSD and significant trauma has become the passion and journey of my life. In 1966, after flunking out of college, and then rapidly getting a 1A draft designation, I joined the Air Force. This was no knee jerk decision. From a very early age, I had been fascinated with aircraft and flying. An 8th grade trip to a local Air Force Base and the airshow that included the Navy's Blue Angels and multiple other demonstrations—and I was hooked.

The journey that ensued was nothing I had planned. Basic training was an experience in reprogramming me from kid to adult, from civilian to military. I maxed the exams the Air Force administered, and after basic training to tech school, I went through almost a year of specialty training as an intelligence analyst, got a top-secret security clearance, and did some very interesting and challenging work.

It meant leaving the U.S. for the first time and adapting to new cultures and new personal challenges. From an assignment in the Philippines, I volunteered in 1968 to go to Vietnam where I spent two years and was discharged in June of 1970 when my four years were up. In Vietnam, I experienced multiple rocket attacks, saw people die, and experienced horrors the mind can never clear but a war zone presents. As an intelligence analyst, I was privy every day with information regarding acts of inhumanity that people render to others. On special duty assignments I got to experience firsthand many events that even half a century later still cause nightmares.

One of the activities I was involved in with my unit was volunteering to work with an orphanage operated by Catholic Sisters in Saigon. These were children from murdered families, brutalized villages, and a life that most of us cannot imagine. Spending time with those children, talking with the nuns, and looking at my future, I decided to go back to college, seriously this time.

I was now motivated with a desire to make a difference after what had been imprinted on my soul. That was my plan. But what I didn't plan for was the experience that as a Vietnam Veteran I found upon returning home. After several *"learning experiences"* with the attitude toward veterans in the 1970s, I learned to keep my mouth shut, dig into school, and by 1975 had my BA, a master's degree, and an entry into the mental health field.

Twenty years later, I managed to obtain a PhD in counseling with a focus on trauma, suicide, and cult psychology, co-authoring a book regarding individuals who underwent ritualistic abuse and severe trauma. Some of the individuals I treated at that time surpassed the horrors I had experienced while in a combat zone.

While I enjoyed the work and felt that I had an impact, something was missing. I was drinking heavily and using that as a *"tool"* to numb the pain and the nightmares that often followed. On May 22, 1982, I stopped drinking and resolved to find some answers.

In 1984, I went to a conference in Washington DC. As our bus drove through town, we passed the Vietnam War Memorial, the dark swath cutting through the landscape, delivering the message of over 58,000 names permanently etched on the *"Wall."* A couple on the bus commented how ugly the memorial was, while I was just thankful that my name was not one etched on the surface. Ironically, but typical of most of us vets at the time, no one on that bus knew of my experience even though several were what I called friends who thought they knew me.

In the middle of the night, I woke up and felt a strong need to visit that wall. I got dressed, went out into the night, and without knowing where I was going, felt drawn and after an hour saw the *"Wall"* in the distance. It was then, sitting there staring at the reflective surface, drenched from a thunderstorm, that my healing began, after over 14 years of feeling lost.

Charlie Daniels' song *"Still in Saigon"* describes what many of us did and still do experience. I went home the next day with a case of pneumonia but also with a resolve to do something to make a difference and come out of my self-imposed exile. I began to share, reach out to other veterans, learning and growing in my own journey forward.

In 1986, my family and I moved to Rochester, Minnesota, to be Clinical Director of a faith-based suicide crisis line. As a licensed mental health professional who also had a faith background, the fit seemed perfect to again reach out and help the most vulnerable. The shock came with the multiple calls that my 40 counselors and I received. The majority were severe trauma victims—sexual assault, violence, and abuse in many forms.

Even more significant was the fact that one out of every three calls was from a veteran, often in the middle of night. Tortured souls fitting all of the high-risk suicide indicators of plan, means, and hopelessness.

I learned later this is a condition called *"survivor guilt,"* a special kind of hell that torments in a way that is difficult to imagine. Through those calls I learned, and by the grace of God, managed to get those individuals to more significant help after our call. To the best of my knowledge, we did not lose one person who called during that time.

In 1987, I was asked to speak at a conference dedicated to *"Vietnam and the Women's Experience,"* focusing on two groups. One was nurses who had served in combat, eight of whom have their names inscribed on the Vietnam War Memorial. The second group was spouses and significant others who stayed home, managed families, watched the horrors of war on the evening news.

My assignment as a mental health professional, running a suicide crisis line, and who was also a veteran of Vietnam, was to speak about suicide.

As an almost afterthought the planning team said, "Uh by the way Steve, since you are here and have some experience in presenting, could you also do the opening on PTSD?" I said "sure" but then wondered how I would do that.

As our book explains, PTSD symptomology has existed since the beginning of time, but the official diagnosis did not come into play until the advent of the DSM III in 1980, the psychiatrist guide to diagnosing PSTD. I had heard the term and was somewhat familiar with the criteria, but the area I was working in at the time did not get into the DSM beyond a paper weight on my desk.

To help with my presentation one of the team gave me a booklet from the Disabled American Veterans (DAV) outlining PTSD and how it was different for Vietnam veterans. That book was like looking into a mirror, and many of those unanswered questions as to *"Why"* began to crystallize.

With that open door, my study began moving me up to today. Although I had the degree and license, for the *"whole book,"* to be truly competent I needed to go deeper. Over the next 30 years, I sought out books, seminars, and those veterans who know "*What*" but do not understand "*Why*."

We are told there are 22 or more veteran suicides a day (the actual number may be greater). Many veterans become so immersed in hopelessness that they end their lives. Of those 22 or more a day, I have been told during some of my trauma training that 19 of the 22 never received help, sought it out, or due to the stigma, saw themselves as beyond useless, evil, broken human beings not worthy or capable of help.

In 2021 through my specialization and reputation as a PTSD specialist, veteran, and licensed mental health professional, I met my co-author through a tragic event he has described. He had been tormented by his Vietnam demons for over 56 years, and now was in a situation that pushed him to the limit. Together in my office, the veil was lifted, and the reality set in that he was not crazy or defective but was someone with an injury no different than any other a human can experience.

As a team, we learned—he on this *"PTSD thing"* and me through his incredible thirst for knowledge. Out of that journey came this book whose primary goal is to help others not go through the journey we both had experienced but to turn on the light of hope to help those suffering from similar trauma see and understand that they are not crazy or defective but are the result of an injury that is neither their fault nor is in any way hopeless.

With that mission, these two *"old warriors,"* at age 76 and 87 respectfully, present this book to you, the reader. It is out of that desire that on what may be our last mission and last battle in a fruitful life to give help and hope to those struggling with the torment of PTSD.

This book is the launching pad to put in the hands of those who are suffering from the results of severe trauma and all that comes with it. Our desire, yes, our passion, is to impact that process and give help, hope, and happiness to all that are now struggling.

We are here with all of you until our last breath, and as these pages continue to be read, hopefully long beyond. As brothers and sisters together, we will take on what is often the biggest battle we will ever fight.

Thank you for coming along on this journey with us. We are here.

Dr. Steve Lansing, Sgt. USAF
Rochester, MN
Email: <u>Drsteve@vetsempowered.org</u>

MY STORY – B. WAYNE QUIST

It was not until sometime after the accident on August 31, 2021, that I began to understand PTSD. That night my problem came back overwhelmingly as I witnessed a teenage girl die, blood spurting from her nose and mouth as she took her last gasping breath. I had a full-blown out-of-body, dissociation experience like I had in Vietnam 1965-1968, and Saudi Arabia in the 1980s.

Flashbacks of blood and gore and an "out-of-body" sense of unreality the night of the accident soon brought me into therapy. I learned that I had complex PTSD, untreated for over 50 years. I had coped most of my adult life with alcohol and escaped into 18-hour workdays—reading, writing, historical research, riding the line on my motorcycle, working—with daily beer and wine to dull the pain of dissociation, derealization, and feelings of unreality. I believed I was deranged and had gone crazy. I was terrified to tell anyone, certainly not my commander, not even my wife.

The night of the accident I was arrested and booked into the local county jail. The final accident report by the highway patrol stated I was not the primary cause of the accident; a plea bargain transferred me into Minnesota's Veteran Treatment Court as one of the conditions of my probation. A few days after the accident, I was introduced to Dr. Steve Lansing, a top PTSD therapist and member of Minnesota's Veterans Treatment Court system. Through Steve's expert knowledge and skillful therapy, my eyes were opened to a new world. Steve helped me understand that I suffered from complex PSTD, untreated for over 50 years.

It started for me when an aircraft mechanic was beheaded as he accidentally walked into the moving propellor of an aircraft parked next to mine. Body parts and blood were strewn throughout the area on the parking ramp. My first PTSD "out of body" derealization experience occurred a few days later, after I returned to my home base. I struggled to work my way through the unusual and frightening experience of unreality, distortion, dissociation, and derealization.

It was like a circuit breaker had popped in my brain. I felt detached from myself and my body, as though viewing reality from a distance, out of my body. It was an unbearable feeling that induced panic. I thought I was deranged and going mad. I told no one, not even my wife or close friends; and not the flight surgeon or my squadron commander, for fear of being grounded and taken off flying status. I slowly worked my way out of it by routinely using alcohol as a coping device and never told anyone of the experience, until I met Steve.

During the Tet Offensive and Siege of Khe Sahn in February 1968, I had landed from an "Air Evac" aeromedical evacuation mission at Da Nang Air Base in South Vietnam. Dozens of dead and wounded were lying on the tarmac, waiting to be loaded onto evacuating aircraft. Enemy mortars were exploding on the ramp, and a young marine called out for a cigarette. He said he was from Minnesota, and I said, "Me too." I found a C-ration with a pack of Lucky Strikes, but when I got back to the badly wounded marine, he was convulsing, blood spurting from his nose and mouth. He died in my arms as we moved him.

This was my second "out of body" PTSD experience—derealization, isolation, detachment, dissociation from reality. It lasted several days and would return periodically over the years, made worse by witnessing new trauma or sometimes even by the evening TV news. Over the years, episodes of PTSD derealization would return, triggered by the sight or smell of blood or decomposing bodies and sometimes even by the smallest of things.

During the early 1980s, I was a senior member of an Air Force detachment in Saudi Arabia and guest of the King. Fridays are the Muslim Sabbath. On a Friday morning, shortly after our arrival, I was escorted to downtown Riyadh near the Grand Mosque by senior Saudi officials and forced to stand in the front row to witness the public beheading of a criminal. Blood flowed like a river as the head was quickly severed from the body with a long, sharp, curved sword.

My third "out of body" PTSD derealization experience soon developed. Sleeplessness, nightmares, and flashbacks of prior trauma started within days and continued off and on for years. I was forced to witness a second public beheading by my hosts in Saudi Arabia a few years later and experienced persisting "out of body" PTSD outbreaks that would last on and off for several weeks.

Throughout my Air Force career, especially as I rose into senior ranks with greater authority and responsibility, I became defensive and insecure out of fear my condition would be detected by senior officers and I would be grounded, removed from flying status, and medically discharged. In 1989, I returned to the U.S. after living in Europe and the Middle East for many years.

Desert Shield and Desert Storm (1990-91) made an enormous impact on me because of severe and lasting symptoms of PTSD that were triggered when Iraq invaded Kuwait and the U.S. deployed over 500,000 American and allied troops into Saudi Arabia. I was physically and psychologically disabled for several months and sought medical treatment, but PTSD was never discussed by doctors or Hazelden therapists at the time.

I slowly recovered on my own, digging deeply into historical research and writing. This became my "go-to" remedy, along with alcohol, to counter PTSD and offset recurring "out-of-body" dissociation episodes. I wrote two books following 9/11 and lectured widely on the ideology of Al Qaeda and ISIS, based on many years in the Middle East, following combat support duty in Vietnam from 1964-1968. I could not resist watching beheadings on TV by Islamic State (ISIS) killers in Iraq, Syria, and Jordan, even as disabling "out of body" episodes inevitably returned.

Following the fatal accident in August 2021, and listening to Dr. Lansing at our weekly "Tuesdays at Two" sessions, I looked deeply into my life and long history of persistent "out-of-body" PTSD episodes. Reading dozens of books on PTSD and tracing the history of PTSD in between our weekly therapy sessions, things began to make sense and fall in place. Maybe I wasn't crazy after all, as I had thought for so many years—maybe there was hope, even for someone like me.

I knew a lot about the history of war, combat fatigue, and shell shock from a lifelong study of previous wars, especially ancient Greek history and the American Civil War but I had rejected the upsurge in modern PTSD therapy as "feel-good" stuff for the baby boomer generation, their children, and grandchildren. I was self-assured in my lack of knowledge, but Steve soon had me realize the folly of my ignorance and what trauma actually does to rewire the brain.

Beginning in the 1950s with the marines, and during my Air Force career into the 1980s, nearly all of my Marine Corps and Air Force mentors were battle-hardened World War II and Korean War veterans. It is now apparent that many suffered from after-effects of severe combat fatigue (PTSD). They had been toughened during the Great Depression, and their combat philosophy was simple: "When the going gets tough, the tough get going."

That was how I was trained, what I believed, and why I thought for so long that PTSD was for sissies. Now I know better, but that thinking still exists among some of our leaders today. I never talked about this stuff, not to anyone, until I met Steve.

B. Wayne Quist, Colonel, USAF (Retired), Joe's nephew
Lake City, Minnesota
Cell: 952-270-8764
Email: Colwayne@vetsempowered.org
Website: www.vetsempowered.org

MISSION BIG WILLY-WON

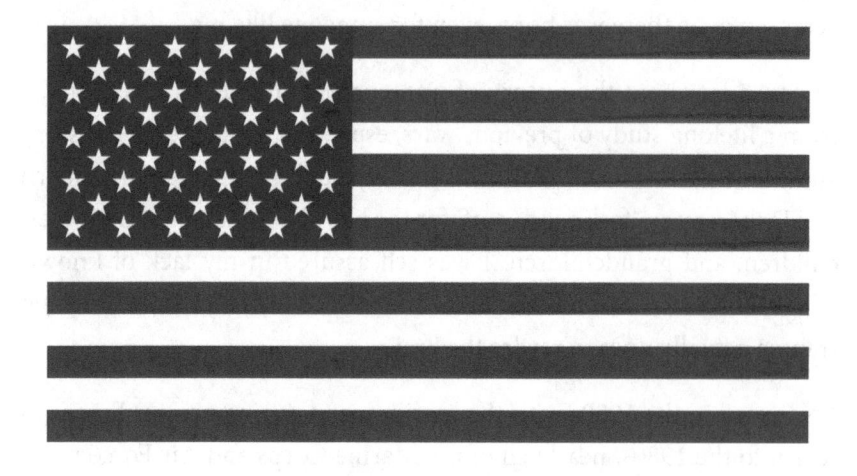

"AND DEATH SHALL HAVE NO DOMINION"

COLONEL B. WAYNE QUIST, USAF (RET)

Senior International Business Executive

Author & Lecturer on American History & Radical, Militant Islamism

"The Triumph of Democracy Over Militant Islamism"

"Winning the War on Terror: A Triumph of American Values"

"God's Angry Man: The Incredible Journey of Private Joe Haan"

"The Millersburg Swedes & the Northfield Bank Robbery"

"Twin Pillars of Terror: Iran vs Saudi Arabia"

"The Trials and Letters of Corporal William Cunningham"

"Dear Donald" and "The History of Christdala"

"Veterans in Crisis: Treating the Unique Needs of Those Who Served, Vol. One and Vol. Two"

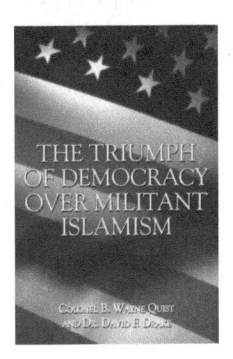

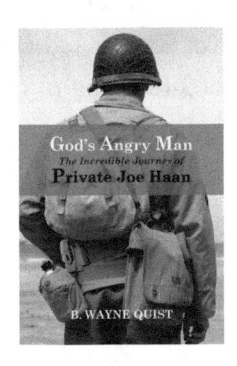

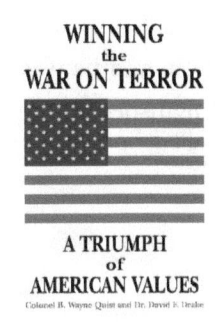

Colonel B. Wayne Quist is the author of publications in the fields of national security, political science, and history and spoke at the 2004 Nobel Peace Prize Forum. After 9/11, he was a popular speaker on the ideology of al Qaeda and ISIS, writing and co-authoring several books and articles. He has a B.A. from St. Olaf College in Northfield, MN, where he grew up, and advanced degrees from University of Southern California and The National War College in Washington, D.C.

Wayne served as a private in the Marine Corps Reserve and entered the Air Force after graduation from St. Olaf. He retired as a full Colonel with 3,500 flying hours, serving in Vietnam, Europe, Middle East, and The Pentagon in Washington, D.C. His Middle East experience began in 1968, and he led a U.S. AWACS deployment into Saudi Arabia following the fall of the Shah of Iran in 1980. Over the years, he has met with numerous heads of state and senior leaders in the region.

After retiring from the Air Force, Wayne lived in Europe and the Middle East heading operations for a Fortune 500 company. Returning to the U.S., Wayne became a partner in an investment banking firm specializing in the sale and recapitalization of privately held companies. He served on the boards of Veterans Empowered Inc, the Christdala Preservation Association, Kierkegaard House Foundation, Center for Democracy and Human Rights in Saudi Arabia (CDHR) in Washington, DC, Lake City Historical Society and Heritage Preservation Commission; and he was the 2003 recipient of the Northfield High School Distinguished Alumni Award.

VETERANS EMPOWERED INC

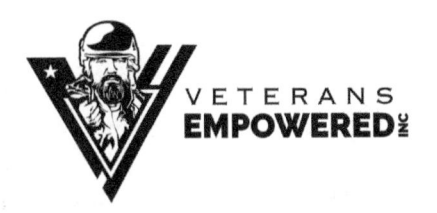

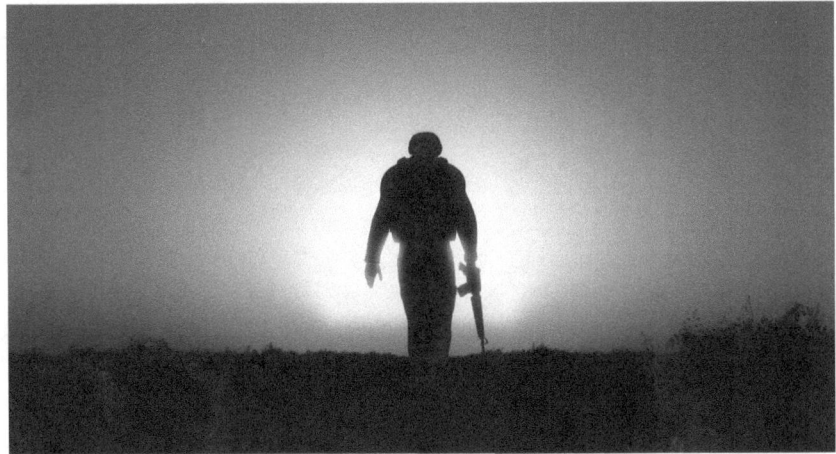

Image by kjpargeter on Freepik

ENDINGS ARE BEGINNINGS